Praise for

The Nurse's Etiquette Advantage, Second Edition

"The Nurse's Etiquette Advantage is a fun, engaging, and enlightening way to learn and refine etiquette that will help enhance professional and personal relationships and propel your career forward. The book accentuates key interactions with our nursing colleagues, physicians, patients, and business associates. Written in a conversational style, it includes essential information in a creative format, highlighting notable quotes, tips, faux pas, good ideas, end-of-chapter FAQs, and take-away tips. This book will give you an edge when you're seeking career advancement!

–Nan Callender-Price, MA, RN
Executive Director, Continuing Nursing Education
OnCourse Learning

"It has been said that you have only one chance to make a good first impression. For a nurse, every encounter is important. Etiquette competency has the potential to make or break a career. Kathleen Pagana's newest edition of *The Nurse's Etiquette Advantage* provides valuable tools for professional interactions. Seldom is there an educational book that is both captivating and entertaining—the format of this book makes it difficult to put down. Make an investment in yourself by gaining skills in professional etiquette that will help you always leave a good professional imprint."

–Carol M. Headley, DNSc, RN, ACNP-BC, CNN
Nephrology Nurse Practitioner, Veterans Affairs Medical Center

"Kathleen Pagana has truly provided a requisite service for all nurses. Her guiding principles regarding handshakes, cocktails, dining, global travel, and other areas assist us in developing better relationships. *The Nurse's Etiquette Advantage* reacquaints us with the niceties of generations past and prepares us to more successfully negotiate the business of healthcare."

–Dennis Sherrod, EdD, RN
Professor and Forsyth Medical Center Endowed Chair of
Recruitment & Retention
Winston-Salem State University

"A must-read for every nurse who wants to be more confident and professional. *The Nurse's Etiquette Advantage* is bursting with career-enhancing information that strengthens business relationships. This book includes take-away tips, etiquette faux pas, and frequently asked questions for every business situation. It is a vital tool for all nurses who desire to move their career forward."

–Nancy Clover, RN, COHN-S, FAAOHN
President, Occupational Health Connections

"Kathleen Pagana has written a necessary and practical guide to help nurses and students at all levels showcase themselves in the best professional light. 'Impression messages' can either promote or derail one's career. This must-read book provides everything you need to know about conveying professionalism in your self-presentation and in interactions with others. It is a fun-to-read road map that lays out the landscape that nurses must navigate to be successful in a nursing career."

–Connie Vance, EdD, RN, FAAN
Professor Emeritus
Consultant, The Mentor Connection in Nursing

"*The Nurse's Etiquette Advantage* is a must-read for all nurses from student to advanced practitioner. Learning and mastering the skills outlined in the book are essential for career and personal success at the highest level, not to mention propelling forward the profession as a whole."

–Donna Cardillo, MA, RN, CSP
The Inspiration Nurse
Dear Donna columnist at Nurse.com

The Nurse's Etiquette Advantage

SECOND EDITION

How Professional Etiquette Can Advance
Your Nursing Career

By Kathleen D. Pagana, PhD, RN

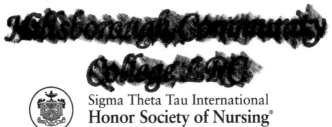

Sigma Theta Tau International
Honor Society of Nursing®

The Honor Society of Nursing, Sigma Theta Tau International (STTI), is a nonprofit organization whose mission is to support the learning, knowledge, and professional development of nurses committed to making a difference in health worldwide. Founded in 1922, STTI has more than 135,000 members in more than 85 countries. Members include practicing nurses, instructors, researchers, policymakers, entrepreneurs, and others. STTI's 496 chapters are located at 678 institutions of higher education throughout Australia, Botswana, Brazil, Canada, Colombia, Ghana, Hong Kong, Japan, Kenya, Malawi, Mexico, the Netherlands, Pakistan, Portugal, Singapore, South Africa, South Korea, Swaziland, Sweden, Taiwan, Tanzania, United Kingdom, United States, and Wales. More information about STTI can be found online at www.nursingsociety.org.

Sigma Theta Tau International
550 West North Street
Indianapolis, IN, USA 46202

To order additional books, buy in bulk, or order for corporate use, contact Nursing Knowledge International at 888.NKI.4YOU (888.654.4968/US and Canada) or +1.317.634.8171 (outside US and Canada).

To request a review copy for course adoption, e-mail solutions@nursingknowledge.org or call 888.NKI.4YOU (888.654.4968/US and Canada) or +1.317.634.8171 (outside US and Canada).

To request author information, or for speaker or other media requests, contact Marketing, the Honor Society of Nursing, Sigma Theta Tau International at 888.634.7575 (US and Canada) or +1.317.634.8171 (outside US and Canada).

ISBN: 9781940446141
EPUB ISBN: 9781940446158
PDF ISBN: 9781940446165
MOBI ISBN: 9781940446172

Pagana, Kathleen Deska, 1952- , author.
  The nurse's etiquette advantage : how professional etiquette can advance your nursing career / by Kathleen D. Pagana. -- Second edition.
    p. ; cm.
  Includes bibliographical references and index.
  ISBN 978-1-940446-14-1 (alk. paper) -- ISBN 978-1-940446-15-8 (epub) -- ISBN 978-1-940446-16-5 (pdf) -- ISBN 978-1-940446-17-2 (mobi)
  I. Sigma Theta Tau International, issuing body. II. Title.
  [DNLM: 1. Nurse's Role. 2. Career Mobility. 3. Interpersonal Relations. 4. Interprofessional Relations. 5. Nurses--psychology. 6. Professional Competence. WY 88]
  RT86.5
  362.17'3--dc23
                              2015012462

First Printing, 2015

Publisher: Dustin Sullivan   Principal Book Editor: Carla Hall
Acquisitions Editor: Emily Hatch   Development Editor: Kate Shoup
Editorial Coordinator: Paula Jeffers   Copy Editor: Kevin Kent
Cover Designer: Rebecca Batchelor   Proofreader: Erin Geile
Interior Design/Page Layout: Rebecca Batchelor Indexer: Jane Palmer

Dedication

This book is dedicated with much love to my husband, Tim, and our three daughters, Jocelyn, Denise, and Theresa.

Acknowledgments

This book would not have been possible without the help, support, and inspiration from so many people. I want to express my special thanks to Marianne P. Deska, Marjorie Brody, and Amy Glass.

About the Author

Kathleen D. Pagana, PhD, RN, is a dynamic speaker and best-selling author. She is an emeritus professor at Lycoming College in Williamsport, Pennsylvania, and the president of Pagana Keynotes & Presentations. She has been a leader in healthcare for more than 35 years. She has a BSN from the University of Maryland and an MSN and PhD in nursing from the University of Pennsylvania.

She is the author of more than 85 articles and 28 books. Her business etiquette articles have appeared in more than 15 different national publications. Her most popular books, *Mosby's Diagnostic and Laboratory Test Reference* (12th ed.) and *Mosby's Manual of Diagnostic and Laboratory Tests* (5th ed.) have sold almost 2 million copies, with translations in French, Chinese, Korean, Greek, Polish, Spanish, and Portuguese.

In her positions as patient care manager, military officer, faculty chair, academic dean, and director on the board of a healthcare system, professional etiquette has helped her handle a number of business challenges. She has enjoyed the privilege of helping thousands feel more comfortable in professional and business situations where they are in the spotlight and need to look and act their best.

Table of Contents

Foreword

Throughout my career, I have focused on enriching the lives of nurses and supporting their retention in the profession. I am delighted to say that the second edition of *The Nurse's Etiquette Advantage: How Professional Etiquette Can Advance Your Nursing Career, Second Edition* supports these goals. Through her research, writing, and speaking experience, Kathleen Pagana has clearly developed a niche for professional etiquette. Better yet, she has taken a subject that is often dry and turned it into a fun and engaging book—I especially like the etiquette quiz, faux pas, FAQs, and take-away tips.

Nurses will find this book beneficial throughout their careers. The chapters on interviewing and professional dress can help nurses get jobs and transition to other opportunities within the profession. Making introductions, remembering names, participating in meetings, using business cards, and handshaking apply to both work and social settings. The networking chapter explains the who, what, when, where, and how of this important art. Networking can happen anywhere and anytime, and the more prepared you are, the more you can benefit.

Pagana also explores the challenge of the "patient experience" as it relates to financial reimbursement and patient satisfaction, including targeted guides for communicating with patients and fostering collaboration with other professionals. Showing respect, being polite, and making others feel valued contribute to effective communication and team building. Eating meals and attending receptions are key aspects of professional interactions. *The Nurse's Etiquette Advantage* helps nurses enjoy these functions without worrying about embarrassing blunders. Learning an easy way to locate your water glass and dinner roll is part of the value and fun of this book. My favorite dining etiquette tip is the BMW (bread, meal, and water). The faux pas are funny but also educational—because, with knowledge, you can avoid these blunders.

Venturing into technology, Pagana furnishes insightful tips that will make you smarter about how and when you use technology. Etiquette principles apply whether you're using email, voice mail, or texting. Your correspondence generates impressions about your writing ability, organization, and professionalism. Abusing technology can be costly to careers. Social media is very popular, but it is a common source of blunders for everyone, including nurses. The book addresses patient privacy and career disasters related to Facebook, LinkedIn, Twitter, blogging, and other types of media. The author provides websites to help nurses learn to use social media and clearly articulates the relevance of social media for networking.

Nurses who travel or hope to travel more in the United States and internationally will find advice, tips, and warnings that could only have been written by a true "road warrior." The author is generous in sharing experiences, offering guidelines, and promoting safety. Whether traveling by plane, train, bus, or car, the reader will find valuable information and strategies to diminish stress and enjoy the travel experience. International travelers will not be caught off guard if they follow the business etiquette tips. The author also recommends websites and books that are helpful for travelers planning to go abroad.

The Nurse's Etiquette Advantage is a book essential to the career success of nurses, whether new graduates or seasoned leaders. This book informs and delights as it provides easy-to-read, practical information not usually learned in school.

–LeAnn Thieman
Nurse, Hall of Fame Speaker, and Author of
Chicken Soup for the Nurse's Soul series

Introduction

Although nursing education has been focused on leadership, management, and professional issues, etiquette has been the missing link for success in the workplace.

This book describes how to get a job, keep a job, and move ahead in a job. It will prepare you to handle awkward and challenging situations that could diminish your confidence, tarnish your reputation, and derail your career aspirations. After reading this fun and enjoyable book, you will be able to interact more effectively in clinical, business, and social settings. You will be amazed at how often you will think, "I didn't know how much I needed to know."

The premise of this book is that everyone can become an expert in etiquette. Further, the better you become at it, the more you will be sought after for opportunities and positions. In these pages, you will find a reality check for those playing (or about to play) the toughest sport of all—survival in a business world that is often unforgiving and highly critical.

Why is etiquette important for nurses? Etiquette is about relationships. Nursing is a career characterized by professional relationships with all kinds of people in all kinds of settings. By using the guiding principles of kindness, consideration, and common sense, professional etiquette can help you initiate new relationships and enhance established relationships. It can guide you in unfamiliar situations and help you know what to expect from others. For example, this book can help you in the following situations:

- Interviewing successfully for a new job or position
- Introducing yourself and others with confidence
- Demonstrating proper handshake and business card etiquette
- Networking effectively on the job and at conferences
- Knowing how to run a productive meeting
- Learning how to create an online persona

- Dressing to mirror your professional image and responsibilities

- Sending a positive impression with thank-you notes and letters

- Using email, phones, and faxes in a courteous and professional manner

- Using social media to further your career

- Dining with confidence in any business or social setting

- Increasing your comfort and self-confidence during business travel

- Appreciating and respecting cultural difference in global interactions

There are no other etiquette books targeted and customized to nurses. This book contains key business-etiquette content with an application to professional nursing. It will help you level the playing field in your interactions with others.

Key Features

Each chapter challenges the reader with a series of *Do you...* questions.

Do you:

Know what to do when you meet a colleague whose name you have forgotten?

Know how to introduce your spouse to your boss?

Have trouble remembering names?

Have a prepared and practiced elevator pitch?

Know what to do if a client ignores your attempt to shake his or her hand?

Wonder when it is appropriate to give out your business card?

A unique feature of this book is its organization in a question-and-answer format. This allows you to target what you need or want to learn or review.

Is there anything that can be done about sweaty hands?

Yes. Spray them with an antiperspirant once a day. This usually takes about 24 hours to become effective. It that does not work, see your physician.

What is a two-handed handshake?

In this situation, one person's right hand shakes the other person's right hand, and his or her left hand is placed on the other person's body. The most common left-handed positions are on the wrist, forearm, bicep, shoulder, or neck.

Tips point out important points for you to remember.

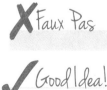

TIP

Never approach someone and say, "Do you remember me?" Be considerate. Put out your hand and state your name.

Faux Pas and *Good Idea!* features provide stories about embarrassing and positive actions, respectively.

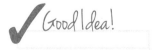

X Faux Pas

✓ Good Idea!

Tables and figures help itemize and illustrate concrete information.

1.1 **Pecking Order for Introductions**

Higher Ranking	Lower Ranking
VP of nursing	New nurse
10-year employee	2-year employee
Father	Daughter's boyfriend
Your boss	Your spouse
Peer in another office	Peer in your office
Client	Colleague

Cultural items are marked with a globe.

Helpful frequently asked questions (FAQs) are included in each chapter.

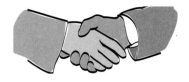

Frequently Asked Questions

? What if I am introducing my boss to my new staff member and I mention the staff member's name first?

Just continue with the introduction and try to remember the proper pecking order the next time. The most important thing about introductions is to make them.

Each chapter ends with
Take-Away Tips.

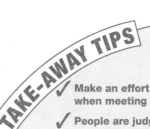

✓ Make an effort to remember names
when meeting people.

✓ People are judged by the quality of
their handshake.

Finally...

"I never knew etiquette could be so much fun," is the most common response of people attending my professional etiquette presentations. The goal of this book is for you to learn (or recall) some career-enhancing material and to have fun at the same time.

You have nothing to lose and everything to gain by reading this book. The skills you learn can be put into practice immediately for career advancement and lifelong value.

Professional etiquette is not optional for personal or professional success. It is a necessity. You can benefit every day in clinical, business, and social settings by using *The Nurse's Etiquette Advantage* to come across as polished, confident, and professional.

1

Making Your Acquaintance

Handling Introductions

Do you:

Know what to do when you meet a colleague whose name you have forgotten?

Know how to introduce your spouse to your boss?

Have trouble remembering names?

Have a prepared and practiced elevator pitch?

Know what to do if a client ignores your attempt to shake his or her hand?

Wonder when it is appropriate to give out your business card?

These are concerns that can add to the stress of any situation where you are meeting and greeting new people. Who hasn't felt awkward during an introduction? You will feel and act more confident if you understand the basic guidelines, and you can improve your interactions with others by practicing these tips for making introductions and creating a positive first impression.

"Civility costs nothing and buys everything."

—Lady Mary Wortley Montagu

Introductions

Does it really matter who is introduced to whom in an introduction?

Yes, it does. There is a pecking order to introductions. The person of honor is mentioned first, and the other person is introduced to him or her. The person of honor is the higher ranking person in the organization. For example, suppose a new graduate is being introduced to the vice president of nursing at a hospital. The vice president of nursing is mentioned first, and the new nurse is presented or introduced to him or her.

What are the key steps of an introduction?

Introductions have three steps.

1. Mention the name of the person of honor first.

2. Say the name of the person being introduced and mention something about him or her.

3. Come back to the person of honor and say something about him or her.

Here is an example of a proper introduction, following these three steps:

> "Theresa, I would like to present Ryan Deska. Ryan is our new staff nurse with 3 years' experience in orthopedics. Theresa Williams has been our VP of nursing for the past 5 years."

Sometimes, when you introduce two people, you will want to facilitate a conversation between them. Here is a way to facilitate conversation after an introduction, using the preceding example:

> "Theresa, I would like to present Ryan Deska. Ryan is our new staff nurse with 3 years' experience in orthopedics. He is also a marathon runner. Theresa has been our VP of nursing for the past 5 years. She is training for her first marathon."

If you are not sure about the pecking order when making introductions, Table 1.1 can help.

1.1 Pecking Order for Introductions	
Higher Ranking	*Lower Ranking*
VP of nursing	New nurse
10-year employee	2-year employee
Father	Daughter's boyfriend
Your boss	Your spouse
Peer in another office	Peer in your office
Client	Colleague

When should I introduce myself?

Always be ready to introduce yourself. None of us is a famous movie star with face and name recognition. Don't stand next to someone, waiting to be introduced. The person you are expecting to introduce you may have forgotten your name. So, to avoid embarrassing him or her, just introduce yourself. Put out your hand and say your name. For example, say, "I don't believe we've met. I'm Denise Miller." Or, "Hello, I'm Denise Miller, and I am a nurse in Same Day Surgery." The other person should return your greeting and introduce himself or herself. If he or she does not give a name, say, "And your name is?"

TIP

Never approach someone and say, "Do you remember me?" Be considerate. Put out your hand and state your name.

What should I do if I go blank and cannot remember someone's name when making an introduction?

This happens. Be honest about it. You can say, "I'm sorry, but I've forgotten your name." Or, "Excuse me, but I'm blanking on your name."

One of my colleagues has asked me to introduce her via email to a contact of mine. Any tips?

In this digital age, you will start seeing a lot more of this type of request. To handle it, send an email to your contact that talks a little about your colleague and why he or she would like to connect. Copy the email to your colleague, who should then follow up with your contact.

Do you have any suggestions for introducing myself and connecting on LinkedIn?

I think the most important thing here is to personalize the request for connecting, especially if you do not know the person. Tell the person why you are asking to connect. For example, you might name a mutual friend who suggested the connection.

Elevator Pitch

What is an elevator pitch?

An elevator pitch is a short speech that sells an idea, markets an individual, or promotes a business. The term is a metaphor for when you gain unexpected access to someone to whom you would like to sell an idea or proposal. Essentially, you should be able to explain a business proposal in an elevator in the time it takes to ride a few floors. A great elevator pitch describes and sells an idea in less than a minute. Of course, it is not restricted to elevators.

What is the desired outcome of a good elevator pitch?

With an elevator pitch, the goal is to capture someone's attention so you can move to the next step—a referral, a follow-up call, a meeting, or a partnership.

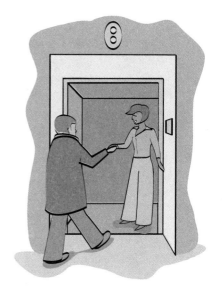

Why would a clinician need an elevator pitch?

The ability to sum up your service or expertise in a unique way is fundamental for any professional. When someone asks you what you do for a living, a well-planned elevator pitch can make the listener's ears perk up and want to know more. Here are some examples of when a good elevator pitch would be helpful:

- When attending a recruitment fair and hoping to get an interview at a certain medical center

- When finishing a degree and hoping to be considered for a new position

- When writing an article and hoping to present the topic at a conference

- When planning to expand a consulting service

What are the key components of an effective elevator pitch?

To write an effective elevator pitch, you must know yourself, what you can offer, and what benefits you can bring. For example, perhaps you are an expert in professional communication and know strategies that you can teach others to foster a better workplace environment.

Follow these guidelines for your elevator pitch:

- **Keep it short:** Limit your pitch to 60 seconds.

- **Have a grabber:** This could be a question, gesture, statistic, anecdote, or personal experience intended to capture or grab the listener's attention and pique his or her interest.

- **Demonstrate your passion:** Your energy will help sell your proposal.

- **Make a request:** For example, do you want to schedule a meeting? If so, ask. The person may be able to give advice about whom to email for further information or whom to contact to set up a meeting.

- **Practice:** Rehearse so that when the opportunity arises, you are ready (Pagana, K. D., 2013c).

Shaking Hands

Am I judged by the quality of my handshake?

Yes, you are. You want to present a confident, firm handshake. Those few seconds you shake hands can weaken or empower a relationship.

The handshake is part of creating a first impression and sending a parting message. Follow these three steps for a proper handshake:

1. Extend your right hand horizontally with your thumb up. Do not cup your hand.

2. Engage a person's hand web-to-web with a firm grip. The web between your thumb and index finger should be touching the other person's thumb web.

3. Shake two or three times and drop your hand.

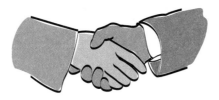

A firm, hearty handshake gives a good first impression, and you'll never be forgiven if you don't live up to it.

—P. J. O'Rourke

See Table 1.2 for tips on handshake etiquette.

(1.2) Handshake Etiquette	
Do	**Don't**
Stand up.	Remain seated.
Make eye contact.	Shake with limp, damp fingers.
Offer a firm grip.	Squeeze the other person's hand too tightly.
Smile.	Turn the person's hand over.
Be considerate of personal space issues.	Refuse or forget to shake hands.

Is there anything that can be done about sweaty hands?

Yes. Spray them with an antiperspirant once a day. This usually takes about 24 hours to become effective. It that does not work, see your physician.

What is a two-handed handshake?

In this situation, one person's right hand shakes the other person's right hand, and his or her left hand is placed on the other person's body. The most common left-handed positions are on the wrist, forearm, bicep, shoulder, or neck. The higher the left hand moves up the body, the greater the possibility for manipulation and control. For example, a left hand clasped around the neck may imply intimacy or ownership (Brown & Johnson, 2004).

Coming from someone you have just met, the two-handed handshake should alert you to the possibility of a controlling or manipulative person. However, this may be perfectly acceptable for friendly, long-term colleagues. Table 1.3 lists handshake variations and their possible interpretations.

Handshake Variations and Possible Interpretations

Handshake	Possible Interpretation
Dead fish (cold and clammy)	The person has a passive personality and low self-esteem.
Pull-in (holds onto your hand and moves you)	The person is maneuvering you and wants to place you somewhere.
Hand on top (palm facing down)	The person with the palm facing down wants to be in control.
Finger squeeze	The person wants to keep other person at a comfortable distance.
Twister (grabs your hand and twists it under his or hers)	The person wants you in a submissive position.
Bone crusher (extreme finger squeezer)	The person equates brute strength with power.

(Brown & Johnson, 2004)

Does gender play a role in handshaking?

In the United States, business is gender-neutral. A man or a woman may initiate the handshake. However, at social gatherings, it is often considered prudent for a man to wait for a woman, especially an elderly woman, to offer her hand.

What should I do if someone ignores my attempt to shake hands?

Gently drop your hand back to your side. There are many cultural preferences and sensitivities that affect a handshake. For example, in the Hindu culture, contact between men and women is avoided, and men do not shake hands with women. There also may be physical limitations or sickness issues.

What should I do if the person I am meeting has an injury on his or her right hand or is otherwise unable to use it?

Greet the person and then follow his or her lead. If the person offers you his or her left hand, shake with your left hand.

What should I do if I am concerned about getting germs from shaking hands?

You have two options here. You could say you are getting over a cold and do not want to spread any germs. Or, you could shake hands, keep your hands away from your face, and then (when possible) politely excuse yourself to wash your hands.

 Does handshake etiquette differ in other countries?

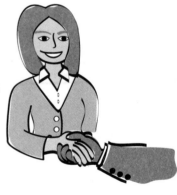

Yes. If you are traveling to other parts of the world, do some research before leaving home. For example, in Germany, a man should wait for a woman to extend her hand for the handshake.

As another example, it may be insulting to a person of Asian descent to look him or her straight in the eye. For more information about international considerations, see Chapter 12, "Going Global."

Remembering Names

I am terrible with names. How can I get better?

Here are some tips for remembering names:

- **Listen carefully:** Often, we are more interested in impressing others than in listening to and focusing on them.

- **Repeat the person's name:** For example, say, "It is a pleasure to meet you, Arlene."

- **Try to connect the person's name to someone:** For example, "Margaret. That is also my mother's name and my middle name."

- **Try to connect the name to something:** For example, think, "Rose has red hair like my rose bushes."

- **Ask the person to spell or repeat his or her name:** For example, say "Do you spell Katharine with a C or a K?"

- **Look at the person's name tag during the introduction:** This will help you remember it, as well as learn how to spell it.

- **Write down the person's name or ask for a business card:** This will help you remember names for the long run.

- **Ask the person for a helpful way to remember how to pronounce his or her name:** For example, when people ask me how to pronounce Pagana, I tell them to think of the word *banana*. Then say "Pah-gann-a" like "bah-nann-a."

Another way to help you remember names is to use the acronym CAR:

- **C**oncentrate on hearing and remembering the name.

- **A**ssociate the name with something or someone.

- **R**epeat the name in your conversation.

What if I met someone before and forgot his or her name?

Say something like, "I met you before. I am not good with names. My name is _____." The other person should say his or her name. Another option is to say, "I remember meeting you, but have forgotten your name. My name is _____."

If someone mispronounces my name, should I grin and bear it?

No. It is a kindness to correct the person right away in a casual and friendly manner. Any delay may add to his or her embarrassment. You could also smile and say, "I've had people pronounce my name many different ways, but the correct way is _____." Your smile implies that you don't take the mistake personally.

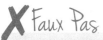 **X Faux Pas**

Dorothy frequently called the medical office of Dr. Nguyen. She pronounced the name "Nu-gen" with a long "U." Several weeks later, she learned from a colleague that the correct pronunciation of the doctor's name was "When." She called the office to apologize and was told that the staff had been getting a good laugh out of this mispronunciation for weeks. She was embarrassed and wished they had been more considerate and corrected her right away.

Business Cards

Do I need a business card?

Yes. Business cards are a great way to capture essential information in a quick and user-friendly manner. Every professional needs a business card for networking.

Patients love having business cards from their healthcare providers. It gives them important contact information.

You can attach a business card to any report or note you send. This lets the person know that you are the sender and provides your contact information.

What information should be on my business card?

That will depend on the purpose of the card. Some basics include your name, degrees, position, and contact information, including your mailing address, phone number, email address, and fax number. If your name is ambiguous (such as *Pat* or *Terry*), use your full name (*Patricia/Patrick* or *Teresa/Terrance*) if applicable, or add a title (for example, *Mr.* or *Ms. Pat Smith*).

If you are trying to promote a service— for example, serving as a writing consultant—make sure that is included on your card. Also include your website if you have one.

Don't cram unrelated information on your card. If you have a side job or hobby, you should have two different cards. For example, your professional information and your cake-decorating business need separate cards (Pagana, K. D., 2006d).

Many nurses include after their names a confusing alphabet soup of letters for their academic and certification credentials. Is this a good idea?

According to Smolenski (2002), this "Campbell's soup approach" can be confusing to the public, other healthcare providers, and nurses themselves. There are basically six types of credentials that can be used after a name:

- Degree (for example, BSN, MSN, PhD, DNS, EdD)

- Licensure (for example, RN, LPN)

- State designation or entitlement (for example, APN, CRNP)

- National certification (for example, RN, C)

- Awards of honor (for example, Fellow of the American Academy of Nursing [FAAN])

- Other certifications (for example, certification for computer skills)

✓ **Good Idea!**

Recently, a colleague asked me if I wanted to run with her in a race to support a cardiac center. When I asked for details, she wrote the website address on the back of her business card and asked me to call her with any questions. Isn't that better than writing on a table napkin?

X **Faux Pas**

Mike was eating lunch at a national nursing convention. At the end of the meal, a new colleague asked him for his business card. Mike took his wallet from his back pocket and pulled out a warm, mushy business card. He quickly learned that his cards were not stored in a professional manner.

For individuals with multiple credentials, Smolenski (2002) recommends the general rule of following the name with the highest credential that cannot be revoked. Then, list in descending order the other credentials from hardest to easiest to be taken away, with awards or fellowships last. To clarify this rule, let's use Janet Swingler, PhD, RN, APRN, as an example. The PhD degree cannot be taken away. The RN licensure could be revoked, and the APRN certification could be taken away if the licensure is lost.

Janet could certainly list additional degrees and credentials if it would help her when applying for a particular position. However, usually only the highest degree is used. It is not necessary to use PhD, MSN, and BSN.

Is it OK to make my own business cards?

Only if that is the only way you will get a card. Homemade cards look homemade. There are websites that offer free cards for a minor shipping charge. Keep in mind that a business card is one of the first graphic impressions of you and your services. Make a good impression with a professional business card.

How should I carry my business cards?

It is best to use a business-card holder or something else that will keep the cards in good condition. A cheap solution is to use a plastic name-tag holder.

Make sure the card you give is in good condition. Don't use a card if it is soiled, bent, or ripped, because the card will not reflect a positive impression of you. It is better to give no card than to give one that is in bad condition.

Develop a system for handling your business cards. For example, keep the cards you give out in your right pocket and place the ones you receive in your left pocket. This will prevent you from accidentally handing out someone else's card.

> **TIP**
>
> **The business card is often described as the handshake you leave behind. Make sure you leave a good impression.**

Is there a proper way to pass out a business card?

Yes. Cards should be presented with the content face up and readable. The receiver should be able to glance at the card and make a comment—for example, "I see you're the clinical nurse specialist in the ICU."

What are some common mistakes that people make with business cards?

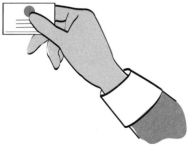

Here are some common mistakes:

- **Passing out your cards as if you are dealing a deck of cards:** You want to be asked for your card. To achieve this, ask for the other person's card first. He or she will most likely ask for yours in return.

- **Writing on someone's card without asking permission:** In some parts of the world, such as Japan, the business card is viewed as a representation of the owner. You deface the card if you write on it without permission.

- **Not having your cards with you:** You never know when someone will ask for your card. Keep them with you at all times. If you are caught without your card, you can send your contact information by a text message or email.

- **Not having a card and asking for someone else's card to write on the back:** This is rude. Jot your information on a piece of paper (Pagana, K. D., 2007a).

X Faux Pas

Karen was relaxing in the hotel lobby after attending a conference in Los Angeles. She met another nurse, Betty, who was in the process of setting up an ambulatory surgery center. Betty asked Karen for a business card. Karen did not have her cards with her, so she asked for one of Betty's cards, crossed out Betty's information, and wrote her contact information on the back of the card. Karen did not realize that this was rude.

 Does business-card etiquette differ around the world?

Yes. If you will be traveling in a foreign country for business, do some research on business-card etiquette before leaving home. People in some countries, such as Germany, are impressed by education and like to see all degrees and titles above the bachelor's degree. In Saudi Arabia, the card should be printed in English on one side and Arabic on the other. When traveling to Poland, bring plenty of cards and give one to everyone you meet (Pagana, K. D., 2006d).

Note also the way business cards are presented. This differs around the world. If someone presents you with a card, follow the person's lead when presenting your card.

✓ Good Idea!

Recently, a new family moved into our neighborhood. As they met the neighbors, they gave everyone a business card with their names (parents and children), address, and phone number. What an impressive way to meet new neighbors and be remembered!

Frequently Asked Questions

What if I am introducing my boss to my new staff member and I mention the staff member's name first?

Just continue with the introduction and try to remember the proper pecking order the next time. The most important thing about introductions is to make them.

What should I say about myself when I introduce myself?

This depends on the situation. If you are meeting someone in a work-related setting, mention your position in the organization. If it is a social situation, mention something pertinent to the setting. For example, if you are at a neighborhood party at Mike's house, you might say, "My name is Ella Gaul. Mike is my next-door neighbor."

What should I do if I forget the name of someone I need to introduce to another person?

One answer is to introduce the person you already know. For example, say, "I'd like you to meet Donald Smith." This will usually result in the third person introducing himself or herself. Alternatively, you can say, "I'm sorry, but I've forgotten your name." Then, make the introductions.

My manager and I will be riding together in the car to a lunch meeting at our branch campus. Is this an appropriate time to bring up a proposal I have been thinking about?

Yes. This is the perfect opportunity to use your elevator pitch. Hopefully, you can capture the manager's interest and plan a follow-up discussion.

 I have heard that it is a good idea to be the last one to release your hand from a handshake. What do you think?

Some experts consider the pause at the end of a handshake a key ingredient of a successful handshake. Pausing demonstrates confidence and expresses sincerity and openness.

 Should a man wait for a businesswoman to extend her hand first for the handshake?

Not anymore. American business is now gender-neutral. However, in a social setting, a man often will wait for a woman to extend her hand first. Handshaking etiquette is different in other cultures.

 What do I do if I am being introduced to someone and that person sneezes into his or her right hand and then extends that hand for a handshake?

You can shake their hand and then go to the restroom and wash your hands. People often refer to this as "taking one for the team." Or, you can say you are getting over a cold and would prefer not to shake hands.

 What do you think of having more than one business card?

This is a great idea if it will help you target your business to a specific audience. For example, if you are a part-time freelance writer, it would be great to have a card related to that—one that is separate from your main job.

Is it OK to use up my supply of business cards if some of my contact information has changed?

Only use them as a temporary measure while you are waiting for your updated ones. Then, throw away the outdated cards. Next time, arrange to get new cards before your information changes.

Is there any way to personalize my business cards?

Yes, business cards can benefit from a personal touch. For example, you might add your cell-phone number on the back if you are hard to reach when traveling. It is a thoughtful gesture that will be appreciated.

What do I do with the business cards I collect after an event?

On the back of the card, note where you met the person and any pertinent information that you want to remember. Also add the date. If you have a lot of cards, photocopy them on one or two pages. Write the date and event name on the top of the paper. Some people have a card reader and enter them electronically into a database.

Cards can also be placed in storage sheet protectors with slots for business cards. These business card pages can hold 10 cards on a side, and can be put into a binder. If you only put one card in each slot, you can read any pertinent information you wrote on the back of the card.

What should I do if someone does not have a business card, and I would like to have his or her contact information?

Take one of your business cards and cross out your information on the front. This will prevent you from accidentally giving this card to someone else. Then write the other person's contact information on the back.

I recently graduated after a long climb up the ladder. As a result, I have obtained many degrees and licenses (LPN, RN, AA, AS, BSN, MSN). What should I include after my name when giving a presentation?

Put your highest degree and your professional licensure after your name. The highest degree assumes the prerequisite degrees. For example, I would use "Deborah Tooney, MSN, RN" or "Deborah Tooney, RN, MSN." If you are speaking to a group of LPNs, you could add the LPN to connect with the audience.

TAKE-AWAY TIPS

✓ Make an effort to remember names when meeting people.

✓ The most important thing to remember about introductions is to make them.

✓ Practice your elevator pitch and be prepared to use it.

✓ People are judged by the quality of their handshake.

✓ The handshake is the only socially acceptable form of touch that can be used in a business situation without raising eyebrows.

✓ A business card is sometimes described as "the handshake you leave behind."

✓ Present your business card with the content face up and readable to the recipient.

✓ The person who receives a business card should look at it and make a comment.

2
When Talk's Not Cheap

Conversations and Networking for Career Success

Do you:

Know how to start a conversation during a networking opportunity?

Need to improve your listening skills?

Wonder if a certain topic is safe to bring up?

Know the proper placement of a name tag?

Know how to gracefully exit a conversation when it is time to move on?

These are concerns that most people have in networking situations. Unfortunately, with today's emphasis on electronic communication, we have neglected some of our interpersonal skills. This has weakened our confidence and skill in face-to-face communication. As an example, think of going to a gym. Note the number of people with earphones. They do not even say "hello" to others.

The ability of nurses to connect with colleagues, clients, and co-workers is essential for success. Read on for some tips designed to make you more confident and professional both at work and in social situations.

Conversational Topics

What topics are safe for conversation?

When you are making new acquaintances within a professional setting, avoid controversial topics. See Table 2.1 for a list of safe and taboo conversational topics.

2.1 Conversational Topics	
Safe	**Unsafe**
Weather	Politics
Sports	Religion
Traffic	Salary or cost of items
Travel	Jokes of questionable taste
Movies and books	Medical problems
Current events	Gossip
Education	Personal misfortunes
New developments in science	Controversial issues

Is it OK to talk about children?

Yes—to some extent. If people ask about your children, answer briefly. Feel free to ask about their children. Be careful to avoid monopolizing the conversation by talking about all the great things your children are doing. Be sensitive to the fact that some people may not be able to have children. People without children may also be bored hearing about your children.

What are some attributes of a good conversationalist?

In addition to being polite and truly caring about others, a good conversationalist does the following:

- Shows interest in others

- Keeps abreast of major news items

- Makes good eye contact when speaking

- Pays attention to body language

- Doesn't pre-judge others

- Avoids correcting a person's grammar in public

- Accepts compliments gracefully

- Knows how to pay a compliment

- Addresses everyone in the group

- Does not monopolize the conversation

- Knows how to make a shy person feel included

- Knows how to ask questions without prying

- Steps in to fill an embarrassing void in the conversation

Your listeners won't care how much you know until they know how much you care.

–Anonymous

The Art of Small Talk

Is small talk really important?

Yes. Small talk is an easy way to start conversations until you find a common area of interest or until business begins. It is used to break the ice and to make people feel comfortable. Small talk is a gateway to new relationships and is also important for maintaining established relationships. There is nothing small about small talk (Pagana, K. D., 2009b)!

X Faux Pas

Marlene was interviewing for a faculty position. As part of her tour around the campus, she was guided by Janet through the library. Marlene made no comments and did not ask any questions throughout the tour. Her responses to Janet's questions were all one-word replies. When the dean met with Marlene, the 45-minute scheduled interview was completed in 15 minutes. Her awkwardness was readily observable. She was uncomfortable and made the interviews uncomfortable. All of Marlene's evaluations were negative, and she was not offered the position.

One always speaks badly when one has nothing to say.

–Voltaire

Do you have any tips for breaking the ice with small talk?

Yes. To aid your conversation, use the acronym OAR:

- **Observe.** Make an observation. For example, "It looks like there are 500 people here."

- **Ask.** Ask questions. For example, "Is this your first time in San Diego?"

- **Reveal.** Reveal something about yourself. For example, "This is my fifth time attending the Sigma Theta Tau convention."

Practice this technique. You can do this anytime and anywhere. For example, you can be standing in the cafeteria line with a colleague, waiting for a meeting to begin, or chatting with the grocery store clerk at checkout (Pagana, K. D., 2013a).

Networking

How important is networking for career development?

Networking is about forming relationships. It is essential for career development because these relationships can benefit you, the other person, your careers, and your lives. These relationships connect you with new colleagues, new opportunities, new information, and different professional practice settings. Think of networking as part of your career, not an add-on if you have time (Pachter, 2013).

Don't make the mistake of thinking that networking occurs only in a professional setting. It can happen anywhere—on the train, at an art class, in the gym. You might be chatting with someone who knows a key person who can help you obtain your next position.

Networking is also facilitated by social media, such a LinkedIn. See Chapter 7, "Avoiding Blunders with Social Media," for more details.

✓ *Good Idea!*

Eloise flew to Chicago to interview for her dream job. While eating lunch, she was chatting with the waiter about her reason for coming to Chicago. To her surprise, the waiter's father was the person she was scheduled to interview with the next morning! She learned a lot of key information that made her interview a great success.

What are some ways to expand my network?

There are several ways to expand your network. Here are a few tips (Pagana, K. D., 2013a):

- Join professional organizations.

- Attend professional meetings.

- Use social media, such as LinkedIn.

- Join a health club or gym.

- Serve on committees and boards.

- Volunteer in your community.

✓ *Good Idea!*

Kim was a new employee in a large company. She joined the company soccer team and met many new friends. She volunteered to help coordinate the holiday party. During the party, she was the master of ceremonies and introduced all the company officers at the party. This was certainly a great way to network and meet all levels of people in a new position.

How can I prepare for a networking session at a conference?

Networking is a powerful way to make new contacts and form new professional and personal relationships. Prepare by being well-read. Read newspapers, magazines, and key journals related to your conference or specialty. Find out who is going to be there and plan to meet at least several new people. Also research people online. This is a great way to find out what they have done and any common interests.

I've learned that people will forget what you said, people will forget what you did, but people will never forget how you made them feel.

—Maya Angelou

X Faux Pas

Donna, the executive director of a nursing association, was the closing presenter at the annual state conference. She spent the day in her hotel room working on her presentation and checking her email. Unfortunately, she missed hearing and meeting the other invited speakers. The conference-planning team wanted to invite one of the speakers to present at the national convention. Unfortunately, Donna was unable to provide any feedback because she had missed the chance to network with the other speakers and attendees.

What is the key to "working the room" at a business or social event?

The key is to demonstrate respect, courtesy, and consideration for the feelings of others as you stay alert for networking opportunities. Good manners are good for business, and bad manners may mean no business. To paraphrase the great Maya Angelou, we may forget what people say to us, but we remember how they made us feel.

> **TIP**
> If you can spot someone "working a room," that person is doing it wrong.

Working the room does not entail flitting from person to person, handing out your business cards, and pumping hands with as many people as possible in a short period of time. If you don't care about people, they will easily sense your insincerity.

How do I work the room?

The easiest person to approach is a single person standing alone. That person will appreciate your walking up and introducing yourself.

If you see couples, take note if they are in an open or closed stance. If they are in an open stance (standing side by side), feel free to approach and introduce yourself. If they are in a closed stance (standing face to face), this implies they are having a private conversation. Don't approach them.

Closed Stance   Open Stance

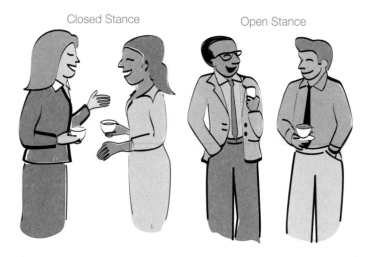

With groups of three, note the open or closed standing positions. Approach a group with the open stance. If you observe a large group of four or more people standing in a circle, that group is closed.

There are basically six ways that people assemble at a networking event:

- Standing alone
- The open two

- The open three

- The closed two

- The closed three

- Larger groups standing in a circle

The first three types of groups will generally be welcoming. Avoid the latter three unless you know someone in the group (Kintish, 2006).

What should I say as I approach a person or group that I do not know?

Smile and say, "Hello, may I join you?" Then introduce yourself and use small talk to get acquainted.

What do I do if I hear myself talking too much?

You do not want to monopolize the conversation. You can demonstrate your interest in others by letting them speak. Remember the old adage that you were given two ears and one mouth for a reason. You want to listen more than you speak. Here are two acronyms to keep you on track (Kintish, 2006).

- **WAIT:** Why Am I Talking?

- **STALL:** Stop Talking And Listen and Learn

Table 2.2 lists common networking mistakes and how to avoid them.

TIP

Even when you are a guest at an event, act like a host. When you think like a host, you act in a different way. You will be more confident, purposeful, and certain.

Common Networking Mistakes and How to Avoid Them

Networking Mistakes	Tips to Avoid Mistakes
Skipping the networking reception at a conference	Arrive early to mingle with other guests or the speaker.
Approaching the event with a negative attitude	Approach the event with enthusiasm.
Focusing on your personal agenda	Try to be a resource for others.
Forgetting your business cards	Always carry your business cards with you.
Not writing down pertinent information	Jot down notes on the back of a business card.
Connecting only with your friends	Expand your network by making new contacts.
Not following up afterward	Schedule time afterward for follow-up.
Drinking too much	Drink responsibly.

What is the best way to handle a compliment?

Smile and graciously say, "Thank you." You could add to this by saying, "Thank you. I appreciate that." Here are some helpful hints for giving or receiving a compliment (Mitchell, 2004):

- Discounting a compliment makes you look unprofessional.

- Don't feel compelled to return the compliment.

- Do not ask where someone bought his or her outfit or how much it cost.

- Do not brag about your designer labels.

- Make sure you are sincere when complimenting someone.

Are there cultural considerations for networking?

Yes. There are many cultural considerations, such as personal space, eye contact, topics of conversation, handshaking, and use of the business card. If you know who will be at a networking session, you should learn in advance about cultural preferences and sensitivities. For example, Chileans stand very close when talking. Chinese people may keep their eyes slightly averted as a sign of respect. See Chapter 12, "Going Global," for more guidelines on global etiquette.

How can I disengage gracefully from a conversation?

This is important when networking, because your goal is to meet several people, not to spend the entire time talking with one person. Here are some tips:

- Excuse yourself and say you are going to the restroom.

- Excuse yourself and say you have to make a phone call.

- Excuse yourself and say you need to touch base with a colleague.

- Say, "It was great speaking to you. I'll let you have some time to speak to others."

- Say, "It was nice meeting you. I hope to see you later."

- Say, "Well, Theresa, it has been nice talking with you. Will you excuse me? I see my roommate over there, and I promised I'd catch up with her."

- Introduce the person to someone else and then excuse yourself as you move away.

- Keep your phone on vibrate at professional gatherings. If it should ring, apologize and move away to talk.

Generational Differences in Communication

Where do I start with generational issues in communication?

A good starting point is to understand that differences exist between people of different generations. These create both challenges and opportunities. Business is all about building relationships. This can be harder when people come from other generations. To begin, identify what generation you belong to, as well as what generation others belong to. Use the following guide (Post, 2014):

- **Veterans:** Born before 1945

- **Baby Boomers:** Born between 1945 and the mid-1960s

- **Generation Xers:** Born between the mid-1960s and 1980

- **Millennials:** Born between 1980 and 1995

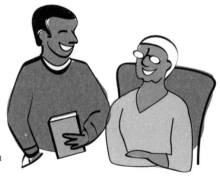

How do I deal with different styles of communication?

Know where people are coming from with their communication style. For example, veterans entered the workforce talking to one another in person; baby boomers communicated by phone; gen Xers use email; and millennials favor texting. Awareness and respect are the keys to working together. This awareness is especially important for nurses, who work with colleagues and clients from different generations.

Veterans may prefer face-to-face interactions. Boomers may prefer face-to-face, telephone, or email. The younger generations prefer electronic communication (Saver, 2011). However, don't assume that all members of the same generation are the same. There are many individual differences.

How do I determine how my colleagues prefer to communicate?

Ask. Alternatively, follow their lead if they initiate the communication. For example, if they sent you an email, respond by email. If they left a phone message, use the phone.

Does multitasking affect communication?

This is an important example of generational differences. The younger generation has grown up texting and doing several things at a time. To the older generation, this behavior seems distracted, disorganized, and often disrespectful. Think about this. Also, don't forget the importance of eye contact when communicating face-to-face.

Mentoring

How can mentoring help with networking and career development?

A mentor can be invaluable, helping connect you to people and opportunities. Listed here are some of the benefits of having a mentor (Vance, 2011):

- Building your confidence

- Increasing your productivity

- Preparing you for leadership roles and other opportunities

- Developing your potential

- Increasing your career satisfaction

When is the right time to look for a mentor?

When you establish your career goals, you will know what you are looking for in a mentor. Target a person with similar personal and professional aspirations.

How long does the mentoring relationship last?

Many of us think of a long-term relationship of mentoring over years or even decades. But according to Vance (2011), mentoring can also include one-minute or instant mentoring.

As a new graduate, I once asked an experienced nurse for help locating something in the supply closet. She not only located the object for me, but went through the entire closet and told me how everything there was used for patients. That one-minute mentorship was invaluable! We can all be one-minute mentors for many people.

Our hospital has an optional mentoring program for new graduates. Should I join?

Absolutely. The first year at work is challenging for new graduates. Having a mentor can help you learn about the hospital from an insider. The mentor can help you deal with challenges and position you to meet your professional goals. Be sure to express your appreciation to your mentor.

Are there mentoring problems that protégés should try to avoid?

Yes. Problems with the mentoring relationship can occur. Here are some to try to avoid (Vance, 2011):

- **Unrealistic expectations:** This can cause feelings of disappointment and betrayal.

- **Power and control issues:** Power should always be used to enhance the potential of the protégé rather than for manipulation or self-aggrandizement.

- **Excessive competitiveness:** This can weaken trust and mutual sharing.

- **Dependence:** After receiving input, guidance, and encouragement, the protégé should make his or her own decisions.

Open, honest communication is the foundation of a healthy mentoring relationship.

Name Tags

What is the proper placement for a name tag?

The name tag should be placed on the right side of your chest so it can be easily seen when shaking hands. When you shake hands, your right shoulder is thrust forward and your left shoulder moves out of the eye line of the other person.

If you are wearing a name tag on a lanyard, adjust the length of the string so it is positioned at the upper part of your chest. It is awkward having to move your eyes from a person's face down his or her body to the navel area to see the name tag. Also, check often to make sure your name is facing out, not flipped over.

What credentials should a nurse in a healthcare provider role wear on a name badge?

At a minimum, a registered nurse should have RN on a name badge. Patients have a right to know who is taking care of them. If you list other letters, it is your responsibility to educate others about the meaning of your credentials.

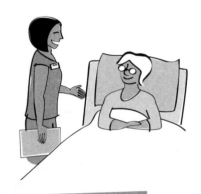

Communicating with a Person with a Disability

Do you have any suggestions for communicating with a person who has a disability?

Focus on the person and not on the disability. Here are some guidelines to avoid offending someone with a disability (Brody, 2005; Mitchell, 2004):

- Avoid using the words *victim*, *cripple*, and *invalid*. *Disability* is preferred over *handicap*.

- Ask if people need help with something before moving to help them. Don't assume a disabled person cannot do something like open a door when in a wheelchair.

- Be prepared to shake hands with a person who has a physical disability. Note which hand the person extends for the handshake and respond in kind.

- Identify yourself as you approach a person who has a visual impairment. Don't raise your voice. If the person has a guide dog, don't pet the dog without asking permission. If the person is blind, make your presence known by speaking and introducing yourself. When initiating a handshake, say something like, "May I shake your hand?" If the blind person initiates a handshake and you cannot shake hands, explain why you can't. For example, say, "I'd like to shake your hand, but I am carrying several packages." Say goodbye so the person knows when you are leaving.

- If you are speaking with someone who has a hearing impairment, stand where you can be seen. Stay within his or her line of vision so the person can see your lips. Reduce background noise. Speak directly to the person, even if he or she has an interpreter present. Add facial expressions. Listen patiently.

- Position yourself at eye level when speaking to someone in a wheelchair. Never assume a person in a wheelchair cannot see, hear, or speak. Don't move a wheelchair out of reach of the person who uses it. Push a wheelchair only if the person wants your help.

How can I ensure successful interactions with deaf and hard-of-hearing patients?

To ensure successful interactions with deaf and hard-of-hearing (HOH) patients, HOH patient and educator A. Kay Tyberg recommends the following (personal communication, 2007):

- Deafness is an invisible disability. Do not be embarrassed when patients tell you they are deaf or hard-of-hearing (HOH).

- Speak face to face to the patient.

- Deaf and HOH patients can do only one thing at a time. So, for example, if weighing the patient on a scale, do not ask other medical-related questions.

- Not every deaf or HOH patient is a skilled lip reader.

- It is inappropriate and rude to use the term *deaf and dumb*.

- Healthcare personnel should wear their name tag in the upper chest area so patients can immediately identify their name and credentials.

- Post a sign above the patient's bed indicating that the patient is deaf or severely HOH.

- If the patient is hospitalized, nurses need to communicate to all shifts that the patient is deaf or HOH.

- If the patient rings the call bell, do not respond over the intercom.

- While in the hospital, see if closed caption television is available.

Can I ask family members of a deaf person to serve as interpreters to save expenses?

According to the Americans with Disabilities Act, it is illegal for hospital personnel to ask family members to serve as interpreters to curtail expenses. A sign language interpreter should be provided upon the person's request (Tyberg, personal communication, 2007).

What is the best way to get the attention of a deaf person?

Physical touch is the normal way of getting the attention of a deaf or HOH patient. Tap the person on the hand, arm, or shoulder to get his or her attention.

Nurse-to-Nurse Collaboration

What are some tips for nurse-to-nurse communication?

Civility is the key word for nurse-to-nurse communication and interaction. Civility is demonstrated in a clinical setting by nurses being courteous and polite with each other. Their conduct should consistently show respect for others, make others feel valued, and contribute to effective communication and team building.

Incivility can be described as rude or disruptive behavior that often results in distress (psychological or physiological) for the person targeted. Incivility can progress through a wide range of behaviors, from eye rolling all the way to physical violence (Clark, 2013). Uncivil behavior has a negative impact on nursing job satisfaction and turnover as well as patient safety and outcomes (Lower, 2007). Table 2.3 lists examples of incivility in the workplace.

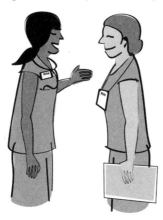

Examples of Incivility in the Workplace

Verbal Abuse	Negative Behavior	Physical Behavior
Making demeaning comments	Humiliating a colleague	Throwing charts
Using condescending language	Scapegoating	Assaulting someone
Making impossible demands	Withholding information	Punching a wall
Expressing impatience with questions	Undermining staff morale	Outbursts of rage
Insulting a colleague in front of a patient	Acting with a cultural bias	Slamming doors
Telling ethnic jokes	Spreading rumors	Banging into others

(Lower, 2007)

Is incivility a new problem in healthcare?

No. It has been around for some time. However, now the healthcare community is making more of an effort to stop it. Here are the three examples of how:

- The Joint Commission has listed incivility and bullying as a sentinel event in 2009.

- State boards of nursing have sanctioned some nursing programs for this problem.

- It would be unlikely for a hospital or medical center to attain or sustain Magnet status if this type of behavior exists.

What are some of the costs of incivility in healthcare?

There are many. Some of the most important are listed here (Clark, 2013):

- Increased stress
- Damaged relationships
- Lowering of self-esteem and morale
- Feelings of vulnerability
- Staff disengagement
- Staff turnover
- Lower productivity
- Decreased safety in the workplace
- Unsafe or compromised patient care

What behaviors promote a positive work environment?

Here are some ideas to promote a positive work environment:

- Greet colleagues with a smile and a "hello" when you arrive at work.
- Offer to help others.
- Thank people for helping you.
- Use polite language and good manners.
- Compliment others when appropriate.
- Avoid listening to gossip.
- Don't be a complainer.

- Respond to phone calls, emails, or other forms of correspondence in a timely fashion.

- Don't interrupt conversations to respond to phone calls, emails, or text messages unless they are urgent. If you must interrupt, ask permission and apologize for the interruption.

- Participate in department events.

- Say "goodbye" to your co-workers when you leave the work setting.

How can I initiate tough conversations dealing with things like tardiness, poor hygiene, bullying, and lack of teamwork?

Before confronting someone with a difficult topic, ask yourself three questions:

- What's the problem?

- How do I feel about it?

- What do I want to be different?

Now you are ready to use the STOP strategy to guide you through difficult conversations. Plan, prepare, and practice this conversation before confronting the person. Here are the components (Pagana, K. D., 2014):

- **State** the situation or problem.

- **Tell** the person what you want.

- **Offer** an opportunity for a response.

- **Provide** closure (review, summarize, or thanks).

What is an example of the STOP strategy?

Here is an example for dealing with a staff member who is tardy:

- **S:** "Monday and Tuesday, you arrived 20 minutes late for work."

- **T:** "I want you to be here at 6:45 a.m."

- **O:** "Can we agree to this?"

- **P:** "Thanks. This will help us work together better."

Nurse-to-Physician Collaboration

How can nurses better communicate and collaborate with physicians?

The key to better communication with physicians is to remember that you are an important member of the healthcare team. Research on Magnet hospitals shows that improved collaboration between nurses and doctors leads to better patient outcomes (Pagana, K. D., 2012b). Here are some tips:

- When you see a physician on the nursing unit whom you do not know, introduce yourself and say, "I am the registered nurse taking care of _____."

- Tell the patient that the physician is on the unit. This will give the patient an opportunity to be ready and in position for an examination before the doctor enters the room. The patient will also have time to think of concerns and questions.

- Inform other nurses taking care of the physician's patients that the doctor is on the unit. This will give them time to organize their questions and concerns.

- Make rounds with the physician and discuss pertinent care issues and needed orders. If you cannot make rounds, have issues documented on a communication sheet.

- If the physician is covering for another physician, provide an update of the patient's hospital course. For example, say, "Mrs. Balon was admitted 3 days ago for syncope. She had a pacemaker inserted 2 days ago and is hoping to be discharged today."

- Check the orders before the physician leaves the unit and clarify as needed.

- If the physician was called to the unit to handle an urgent situation, have the physical assessment findings and updated vital signs available along with the pertinent lab values. Put the patient in a position to be examined. Discuss the concerns that led to the urgent call to the unit.

- If texting a physician regarding a patient, do not use any patient-identifying information. Text a request to talk about a patient and ask the physician to call you.

Why are some nurses reluctant to speak to physicians about patient concerns?

Nurses and physicians are taught to communicate in different styles. Physicians tend to be concise and get to the point quickly. Because nurses are taught not to make diagnoses, they tend to be insecure about presenting their findings and paint a broad picture of the situation when communicating with physicians. Often, physicians become impatient with a lengthy and possibly rambling message (Tocco & DeFontes, 2014).

Are there are guidelines to facilitate effective communication with physicians?

Yes. There are several. I will give two examples. One is the SBAR technique, which is widely used in healthcare (Pagana, K. D., 2012b). SBAR stands for the following:

- **Situation:** What is the reason for your concern?

- **Background:** Why was the patient admitted? What procedures or surgery was performed?

- **Assessment:** What are the vital signs, lab results, and clinical findings?

- **Recommendation:** What would you like the physician to do or order?

For example, suppose you want to recommend an anxiolytic for your patient. Here's how you can use the SBAR technique to convey your recommendation to the physician:

- **Situation:** "Mrs. Collins is complaining of severe anxiety."

- **Background:** "She is 1 day post-op from a lumbar laminectomy."

- **Assessment:** "She is alert and oriented and her vital signs are stable. She has no numbness or tingling in her extremities."

- **Recommendation:** "She said she takes lorazepam 2 mg orally at home when she is anxious. Would you like to order this or something else for her?"

Another technique is the check-back tool for ensuring clear communication and teamwork. This is a concept promoted by TeamSTEPPS and CREW resources. This tool employs closed-loop communication to ensure that information conveyed by the sender is understood by the receiver as intended. Here is an example:

- **Doctor:** "Give me 25 mg of diphenhydramine IV push."

- **Nurse:** "25 mg of diphenhydramine IV push."

- **Doctor:** "That's correct."

What can I do to collaborate better when patient safety is at stake?

Patient safety concerns may require the CUS technique. This is a mutually agreed upon critical language derived from the airlines. For critical language to be effective, all team members must understand it and accept it in a culture that immediately addresses patient-safety concerns. CUS is an acronym for the following:

- **I'm Concerned:** For example, you might say, "Dr. Jenkins, I am concerned about Mrs. Knight. The baby's heart rate is in the low 60s."

- **I'm Uncomfortable:** Here, you could say, "I'm uncomfortable with these late decelerations."

- **This is unSafe.** Finally, you could say, "I don't think it is safe to continue labor."

How can I demonstrate professionalism in a phone call with a physician?

This is a key area for preventing communication breakdown and acting as a patient advocate. Here are some suggestions:

- **Be sure you are contacting the right physician:** The orthopedic surgeon will not want to be called about an abnormal heart rate.

- **Contact the physician by his or her preferred method:** Many physicians use cell phones and do not want to be called on their home phone.

- **Offer specific instructions to unit clerks:** If you are asking a unit clerk to initiate the call, be very specific with your instructions. For example, say, "Please call Dr. Guisseppi at his office and say that I would like to speak to him about the blood sugar on Mike Browning."

> **TIP**
>
> **Open communication improves the quality and safety of patient care.**

- **Be available for quick access when the call is returned:** Make sure the unit clerk can quickly locate you.

- **Have pertinent information at your fingertips:** For example, be ready with the latest set of vital signs, intake and output, assessment data, current intravenous solutions, recent lab reports, medication list, allergy information, and patient chart.

- **Be succinct:** Use the SBAR technique mentioned earlier in the chapter.

- **Be ready to take orders:** Have an order form available and ready to use for phone orders if the physician cannot enter the order electronically.

The Patient Experience

How does communication with patients affect the patient experience?

This is a timely question with healthcare reimbursement. Value-based purchasing is now used to determine the effectiveness of patient care and to determine payment for services. Basically, this is "pay for performance" based on quality of care. The patient experience is one of the four determinants of reimbursement along with outcomes, efficiency, and clinical process of care.

Communication is one of the key components used to evaluate the patient experience. Patient survey questionnaires such as the Hospital Consumer Assessment of Healthcare Providers and Systems (HCAHPS) address core questions about the patient's hospital experience. Examples include questions about communication with nurses, communication with doctors, communication about medications, and discharge information A key component of the patient experience involves listening to patients.

How can I improve my listening skills?

Listening is one of the most generous and gracious human behaviors (Krames, 2002). Never underestimate the power of good listening. A good listener can make the patient feel like the most important person in the world. Table 2.4 lists tips for good listening.

2.4   Tips for Good Listening

Things to Do	Things to Avoid
Make good eye contact.	Finishing sentences for others
Ignore distractions.	Daydreaming
Smile and nod your head.	Interrupting
Ask questions.	Changing the subject
Lean forward.	Looking at your watch or mobile device
Face the person with your body.	Distracting body language (looking around the room)

 Good Idea!

After falling and fracturing his patella, Brian was admitted to the hospital for a patella repair. He started physical therapy (PT) the morning after surgery. After returning from PT, he was upset and told his nurse several reasons why he was unhappy with his treatment by the PT department. The nurse contacted the supervisor of PT and explained his concerns. The supervisor came to the unit to discuss the problems. He was treated by a different therapist in the afternoon and was pleased with the quick response to his concerns. This situation demonstrates the nurse's role as an advocate for patients in vulnerable positions.

What is the best way to respond when a patient thanks you for something?

Smile and say, "My pleasure" or "You're welcome." Don't use the phrase, "No problem." This minimizes the expense, education, and experience it took you to become a professional nurse.

How can networking and conversational tips be applied in clinical settings?

There is a book called *Don't Sweat the Small Stuff.* The advice to not sweat the small stuff does not apply in networking and clinical settings, however. Sweat the small stuff! Small things make a big difference, especially to a client in a healthcare setting. Some guidelines are listed here:

- Address all patients as Mr., Mrs., or Ms. Use a first name or nickname only if the patient gives you permission. Avoid all use of familiarities such as "honey" or "sweetie."

- Greet new patients with the following: "Welcome to _____. My name is [first and last name], and I am the registered nurse who will be coordinating your care until [time]."

- Review the plan of care and treatment goals for the day. Tell the patient the times of any scheduled activities, such as physical therapy. Write this information on a white board, if one is available. Ask for patient input. Don't write anything that would violate HIPAA privacy rules.

- When leaving a patient's room, ask, "Is there anything else you need? I have the time." Make sure the call bell, phone, water, TV, and tissues are within the patient's reach.

Many healthcare facilities are adopting policies and scripting to ensure more positive interactions with patients. See the following sidebar for examples.

Tips for Professional Patient Encounters

- Knock on the door, speak softly, and wait for the patient's permission to enter the room.
- Wash your hands.
- Identify the patient.
- Make eye contact and smile.
- Introduce yourself.
- Provide an explanation of what you are going to do.
- Be gentle in handling the patient.
- Ensure maximum privacy (pull the curtains and close the door).
- Wipe down the needed equipment (such as blood-pressure cuff).
- Do not act rushed even if you are.
- Ask the patient:

    How can I help you today?

    Is there anything I can get you before I leave?

    Do you have any questions?

Used with permission by Ohio Valley General Hospital, McKees Rocks, Pennsylvania

Advice From a Clinical Specialty Area

Because of frequent contact with dialysis clients, nurses may reach a comfort level and disregard the professional boundary lines. Even when nurses are completely at ease with patients, they need to remember that the workplace is not their home. They should maintain a degree of formality and consider the workplace a place of respect. As an example, a colleague recounted a complaint made by her mother, who had recently begun dialysis. The staff in the dialysis unit did not call the mother by her name, but used terms such as "sweetie" and "honey." The patient found this belittling and demeaning. She was an individual with a name. This lax attitude annoyed her and made her uneasy. (Headley, 2007)

Frequently Asked Questions

 What should I do if I am talking with a colleague and someone I do not know joins us?

Introduce yourself. Your colleague may not make introductions because he or she has forgotten your name or the other person's name.

 What should I do if someone keeps asking me questions and never says anything about himself or herself?

Say, "Enough about me. Tell me about you."

 How can I avoid getting drawn into a political or gossipy conversation?

You can say something like, "I've got to go. I have found that politics (or gossip) doesn't mix well in the work environment."

 If a colleague or potential client is unavailable when I call on the phone, how can I find out a good time to call again?

In a polite manner, ask the receptionist, "When do you recommend I try calling back?"

 What should I do if I am having trouble understanding someone who is speaking English as a second language?

Ask the person to repeat what he or she said more slowly. Tell the person you are having a hard time understanding and need his or her help. Put the blame on yourself, not on the speaker. Another option is to call interpreter services to assist.

If I am speaking to someone at a reception, and a friend is waving to me across the room, what should I do?

You can wave and nod, but then return your full attention and focus on the person you are speaking with.

What should I do if I am greeting and meeting people and I need to sneeze?

Have a handkerchief or tissue in your left hand. That way, your right hand will be clean for handshakes.

After I've met someone at a networking session, how can I keep the connection alive?

Make an effort to stay connected. For example, send notes or emails. Try to connect within a week or two so the person will remember you. Call on the phone to say "hello" or to meet for a meal. Acknowledge any awards or honors with a congratulatory note. If you see an article that might interest the person, send it with a brief note.

TAKE-AWAY TIPS

✓ The essence of networking is the building of new relationships.

✓ Respect is a key component of effective intergenerational communication.

✓ Plan a two- or three-sentence response for the inevitable question, "What do you do?" Tailor this to the situation or event.

✓ There is nothing small about small talk.

✓ Try being a one-minute mentor.

✓ If your name tag is hanging on a lanyard, make sure it is turned so it can be read.

✓ Use the term *disability* instead of *handicap*.

✓ Incivility among healthcare professionals can lead to compromised patient care.

✓ Use the SBAR technique to facilitate communication with physicians.

✓ The patient experience is a determinant of healthcare reimbursement.

✓ When calling someone's office, always treat the secretary or receptionist with respect and courtesy.

✓ Make the first move when meeting new people.

✓ When someone tells you that you are a great conversationalist, it is often a compliment to your listening skills.

3

Appearances Are (Almost) Everything

Your Professional Presence

Do you:

Know how to look your best for a job interview?

Wonder why people question what you say?

Think you overdressed for an interview?

Think you made a bad first impression?

Want to look professional in the clinical area?

No matter what some people may say, you are judged by the way you dress. Your clothes are either going to be a positive or a negative factor. Clothes are never neutral. If you are aware of the essentials for professional dress, as well as your body language, you can focus more on what you are saying and doing *without* detracting from your professional presentation.

Clothes and manners do not make the man; but, when he is made, they greatly improve his appearance.

–Henry Ward Beecher

Professional Clothing

Do clothes really make a big difference?

Yes. Suppose you received two gifts. One gift was beautifully wrapped. The other was sloppily wrapped in cheap paper. Which gift would have the greater perceived value? Whether you are interviewing for a job, giving a presentation, or asking for a promotion, the way you dress is an important part of your overall packaging. As with gift-wrapping, the more put together your appearance, the more positive your impression (Whitmore, 2005).

✗ Faux Pas

Elizabeth was seeking a position as speaker for an international communications company. As part of the interviewing process, she was expected to conduct a seminar on presentation skills for business executives. Her speech evaluations were favorable, but the company evaluators made note of her wrinkled suede suit. She was very embarrassed and upset with the feedback about her suit. She had, in fact, been wearing an expensive suede suit that had just been dry-cleaned. This feedback caused her to rethink her professional attire, and she gave away the suede suit and purchased a wool suit.

What judgments do people form about me based on my clothes?

People unconsciously judge your socioeco-nomic status, background, level of educa-tion, and personality based on your clothes (Whitmore, 2005). If you are underdressed, you can embarrass yourself and your col-leagues. If you overdress, you can set the wrong tone and may intimidate others. Be aware that how you dress makes a powerful statement about you.

What impression am I giving if I wear sloppy or inappropriate attire?

Sloppy or inappropriate attire could imply that you do not respect yourself, that you do not place value on appearance, or that you do not care that your appear-ance affects the organiza-tion's image.

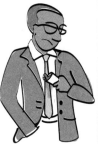

How do I know the appropriate way to dress for different positions?

Look how leaders or managers dress in different positions, and model your attire to match theirs. For example, an educator might have a different profes-sional look than a corporate executive. If you are looking to advance in your career, dress like the people on the next level up.

✓ **Good Idea!**

Jocelyn was delighted to hear that she was the recipient of an award for her work with teens in Washington, D.C. The award was to be presented at a large banquet by a United States senator. Jocelyn was planning to wear a sweater set and slacks until she spoke to her mother. When her mother offered to buy a suit, the matter was settled. On the day of the award, Jocelyn walked across the stage looking confident and stunning in a beautiful suit. Most people walk a little taller and demonstrate more confidence when they wear a suit.

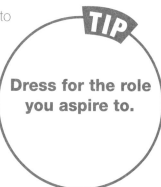

TIP

Dress for the role you aspire to.

Is professional dress more of a challenge for men or for women?

Professional dress is more of a challenge for women. This is because professional dress for men is more easily defined. Men look professional when they wear a suit and tie. The leeway in defining professional dress for women leads to the potential for inappropriate clothing. For example, common complaints about women in a professional setting include tight-fitting and short skirts, unprofessional hair, too much makeup, or clothing that is too casual (Pagana, K. D., 2005b).

TIP

Avoid clothes that reveal too much or leave too little to the imagination.

Why do nurses need to be concerned about their style of dress outside the clinical area?

One of the best features of a nursing career is variety. Not all nurses work at the bedside. There are many nursing positions where business dress is the norm, such as chief nursing officers, hospital presidents, college professors, legal nurse consultants, and board members. Also, when nurses continue their education or change positions, they need to know how to dress for interviewing and collaborating with other professionals.

Table 3.1 discusses professional dress for women, and Table 3.2 discusses professional dress for men.

Tips for Professional Dress for Women

Aspect of Outfit	Tips
Suit colors	Navy blue, charcoal gray, black, burgundy, and taupe are traditional. Wear darker hues during the winter. Wear colors that are flattering to your skin tone.
Suit fabrics	Buy fabrics that wear well. Wool knits, crepes, and microfibers generally wrinkle less. Linens are known for wrinkling.
Blouses	Avoid blouses that are too revealing. If wearing a sleeveless blouse, keep your jacket on.
Scarves	Silk and silk blends hang better than cotton. The classic size is 34 inches square. Scarves can soften a tailored look.
Shoes	The classic pump has a 1½- to 3-inch heel. A spiked heel (3 inches or higher) and flat heels look least professional. Business colors are black, navy, brown, and taupe. Do not wear shoes that are scuffed or have worn-down heels.
Boots	Boots can be acceptable for classic business dress in some settings.
Stockings	Neutral or flesh tones are always smart. Do not wear dark stockings with light shoes.
Belts	The classic width is ½ to ¾ inch. Leather belts should coordinate with your shoes. If metal, match it to other metal (for example, earrings, necklaces, buttons, or a watch).
Jewelry	Your jewelry should accent, not dominate, your outfit. Earrings should be compatible in size to necklaces. Wear one ring per hand. (Wedding and engagement rings count as one.)

continues

Tips for Professional Dress for Women *(continued)*

Aspect of Outfit	Tips
Watches	Match the metal of your watch to your other jewelry.
Eyeglasses	Wear updated frames. Don't let your glasses compete with your jewelry. Match the metal of your glasses to your other jewelry.
Purses	The purse should be neat and functional. A poorly made or worn-out purse can downgrade your outfit. Coordinate your briefcase with your purse.

(Brody, 2005; Post, 2014)

 Tips for Professional Dress for Men

Aspect of Outfit	Tips
Suit colors	Navy blue, gray, and black are the business standards. Dark colors are associated with more authority.
Suit fabrics	Wool is the fabric of choice. The suit surface should be matte, not shiny.
Slacks	Pants fitted to the waist are more slimming. Flat fronts are more slimming than pleats. Cuffs are more classic in style than pants without cuffs.
Dress shirts	White is the dressiest. Shades of blue, gray, tan, and muted green are preferred. A point collar looks fine open or with a tie. Always wear a tie with spread collars.

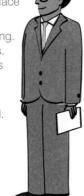

Aspect of Outfit	Tips
Shoes	Shoes should harmonize with the outfit. Wear black shoes with gray, navy, or black suits. Wear brown shoes with tan, brown, or beige suits.
Socks	Match socks with your pants. Exception: With tan pants, socks should match the shoes. Socks should be high enough to cover your shins when sitting.
Ties	Silk is the best fabric. The tie should complement the suit color, but not match it. Wear a wider tie with a wider lapel. Wear a thinner tie with a slimmer lapel. The tip of the tie should end at the top or middle of the belt. Don't wear a tie with a short-sleeve shirt.
Belts	Match the belt to your shoe color. The standard belt width is $1\frac{1}{4}$ inches.
Jewelry	Keep your jewelry subtle and minimal. Do not wear more than one ring per hand. Match metal to metal with jewelry items (for example, gold to gold).
Eyeglasses	Wear updated frames. A round face looks better with square frames. A square face looks better with round frames.
Wallets	Dark leather is the most traditional. The wallet should be thin and not cause a bulge in the back pocket.
Miscella-neous	When wearing a single-breasted suit or sports coat, button the top button when you stand. Unbutton it when you sit down.

(Brody, 2005; Post, 2014)

The apparel often proclaims the man.

–Shakespeare

Do you have any tips for handbags and briefcases?

Yes. These items can detract from your overall appearance if they are shabby and worn. These articles do more than hold important papers, wallets, and cell phones. They hold clues about your professionalism, success, and personality. Think "classic" when purchasing these accessories (Whitmore, 2005).

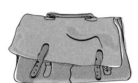 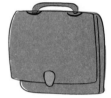

✗ Faux Pas

Jessica purchased a sexy black dress for a cocktail party at her college reunion. She wore the same dress to the hospital's holiday party several weeks later. Unfortunately, she did not project the corporate image needed for the administrative position for which she had just applied. When the committee met to discuss the applicants, several people mentioned Jessica's dress. The bottom line is that what is appropriate for wearing with friends may not be appropriate to wear in a work setting.

How can I put my best foot forward?

Make sure your shoes are in good condition. Dusty and worn-looking shoes detract from a professional impact. Shoes are often assessed to evaluate your attention to detail.

✗ Faux Pas

Roberto was the CEO of a large healthcare facility. He had impeccably good taste and his clothes made a professional impression. However, his wingtip shoes were shoddy. When he crossed his legs, duct tape was visible on the bottom of his shoes. His shoes were an embarrassment to the corporate staff until one brave soul had the guts to discuss his shoes with him privately.

How do I know what colors are flattering for me?

Hold a piece of clothing up to your face and study how you look. A flattering color will make your eye color more intense and your skin tone more vibrant and will give you an energetic look. In contrast, your skin will look sallow, your eyes dull, and your face tired with an unflattering color (Post, 2014). If you're not sure what colors are right for you, consider hiring an image consultant.

What about makeup?

Most women look better with a little makeup. The key is to use makeup to enhance, not to dominate. If you choose to wear lipstick, make sure you don't have lipstick on your teeth.

TIP

Never comment on someone's weight. Even a compliment can be taken in the wrong way.

What about professional women with long hair?

Hair should be kept out of the eyes. It can be tucked behind the ears, pulled back with a barrette, pulled up in a pony-tail, or twisted up with a clamp.

Know first who you are; and then adorn yourself accordingly.

—Euripides

Dressing in the Clinical Setting

What impact does dress have in a clinical setting?

Dress has a bigger impact in a clinical setting than most nurses realize. The way you dress supports or detracts from your professional image. It sends a message to others about how you see yourself and how you want to be perceived by others. It sets the stage for what others may expect from you. Most nurses would agree that they would like to be viewed as professional, intelligent, and competent. They need to ask themselves if their appearance mirrors that image.

If nurses dress too casually, patients may question their attention to detail and their professionalism. Patients often associate appearance with trustworthiness and ability. Does a nurse dressed in bunny print scrubs establish immediate trust, authority, and credibility? Many patients complain that everyone in a clinical setting looks the same. Patients want their nurses to be clearly identifiable. This identification is also essential for having positive interactions with families, physicians, and other members of the health team.

Nurses in White

If you are a patient at St. Clair Hospital in Pittsburgh, Pennsylvania, you can clearly identify your nurse. Nurses wear white uniforms or white scrubs. Nurse aides wear white bottoms with green tops. Joan Massella, chief nursing officer, said the change was done for two major reasons. First, it was done because many nurses did not appear professional due to their style of dress. Second, it was done to improve patient satisfaction. Most patients were elderly and could not differentiate nurses from other hospital employees. Do the nurses like the change? According to Joan, not all of them are happy, but they look great. Do the patients like the change? Yes, the patients and their family members like being able to identify their nurses.

Can scrubs be part of a professional image?

Many hospitals are re-evaluating their dress codes. Randomly selected scrubs in various colors and print designs may be on their way out, as the credibility and professionalism of healthcare personnel are under scrutiny.

According to image consultant Sandy Dumont (personal communication, 2007), uniforms are necessary for professional identification. In her opinion, nurses look most professional when wearing white. She believes that hospitals need to mandate dress codes. If they permit scrubs, she asserts that there should be uniformity. All nurses should wear the same color, so it doesn't look like someone was hired off the street and doesn't have a uniform yet.

Notes from an Image Consultant

In a hospital setting, things are often a matter of life and death, and you show up wearing "pink pajamas" with cartoon motifs. How is a patient to know that you're not there to change the bedpans? Nothing about your appearance announces that you are a highly trained expert who is a member of an honored profession.

Imagine you're boarding an airplane. If the co-pilot greeted you wearing a polo shirt and khakis whereas the pilot wore the traditional uniform, would you be taken aback? Would you assume that the casually dressed pilot was still in training, or that perhaps he was called in to fly at a moment's notice? "Hope he wasn't drinking the night before," you might say to yourself. Furthermore, what would you think about an airline that permitted pilots to dress for their own comfort rather than wear a proper uniform?

Don't cheat your patients of their expectation to be cared for by a highly trained expert who is a member of an honored profession. If you are proud of who you are and what you do, shout it to the world by *looking* like a nurse!

Sandy Dumont is an image consultant with 30 years of experience. She conducts workshops and seminars throughout the country and abroad. Contact her at her website, www.theimagearchitect.com.

Many healthcare systems now have mandated colors for nurses and other professionals. For example, in some hospitals, nurses wear navy blue, physical therapists wear green, and respiratory therapists wear blue. When the hospital logo is embroidered on the neatly pressed scrub top, the look is professional.

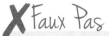

X Faux Pas

As part of hospital orientation, a group of nursing students was told about the hospital and university dress code policy. On clinical days, they were to wear their uniforms and lab coats. But, while pre-planning, they could wear business casual clothes with their lab coats and name tags. One week later, two of the students arrived for pre-planning wearing soccer shorts, tee shirts, and flip-flops. They were not permitted on the unit, and the negative impression they left stuck with them. The staff referred to them as the "soccer girls" for the rest of the semester.

What are some general guidelines for dress in a clinical setting?

All nurses in all settings should look neat and professional. Uniforms, lab coats, and scrubs should be wrinkle-free. Shoes should be clean. Long hair should be pulled back and out of the face. Name tags should be visible and readable.

Body Language

What impact does body language have on the overall impression a person makes?

We all communicate with each other visually, vocally, and verbally. The professional impression you provide is based on the words you use (verbal), the way your voice sounds (vocal), and what people see (visual). The visual element has the strongest impact and consists of everything people see when they look at you. This includes your dress, grooming, and body language.

The care and time you invest in your appearance and words can be undone by body language. For example, suppose you are dressed in a professional manner, but you are slouching and leaning back in your chair. You are probably sending a message that you are not as interested as you should be.

Avoid looking at your watch when talking with patients. This may suggest you have something better to do. Also, when you enter a patient's room, try not to drag your feet, implying you are tired. The patient may feel uncomfortable asking for help.

✓ Good Idea!

Kristin was teaching a workshop on time management. The workshop was videotaped so it could be shown for evening- and night-shift personnel. When Kristin viewed her tape, she was disappointed. She had an unpleasant look on her face, and her posture was poor. Her body language detracted from her professionalism. She used this feedback in a constructive manner and greatly improved her presentation skills. Most people would benefit by critiquing themselves on videotape.

When the eyes say one thing, and the tongue another, a practiced man relies on the language of the first

–Ralph Waldo Emerson

How can I tell if my body language is having a negative impact on my professionalism?

Tune in and be aware of what image your nonverbal communication is projecting. Many negative aspects of body language are bad habits that can be corrected with awareness. Get feedback from others. Table 3.3 offers several body language tips.

3.3   Body Language Tips

Topic	Tips
Standing	Stand tall with your shoulders back and your chin up. Keep your shoulders relaxed. Avoid slouching, swaying, and shifting your feet. Don't keep your hands in your pockets. Folding your arms may denote defensiveness or disagreement. Don't put your hands on your hips.
Sitting	Sit up straight. Cross your legs at the ankles. Avoid slouching. Don't jiggle your knees or tap your feet.
Facial expressions	A sincere smile denotes warmth and friendliness. A false smile makes you look phony. A frown makes you look angry or worried. Be animated, but don't overdo it.
Eye contact	Looking at the eyes of another shows your interest. Occasionally look away and move your eyes to another part of the face. Don't stare or shift your eyes.
Movement	Move with confidence and purpose. Don't drag or shuffle your feet.
Gestures	Use gestures to make a point. Vary your gestures. Gesture with open hands. Don't wring your hands, point, or make a fist. Don't overdo gesturing.

(Pachter, 2013; Post 2014)

Also, avoid the following:

- Playing with your hair or jewelry
- Biting your lips
- Twisting your mustache
- Drumming your fingers
- Clicking pens
- Picking your teeth
- Biting your fingernails
- Jiggling keys or change in your pocket

Frequently Asked Questions

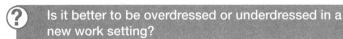

Is it better to be overdressed or underdressed in a new work setting?

In general, it is better to err on the more formal side. Remember, you can always remove a jacket, but you cannot put one on if you didn't bring it with you.

If I am dressed inappropriately, couldn't it mean that I just did not know any better?

Yes. But that is not an excuse. You need to find out the appropriate dress. By your inappropriate dress, you could also be suggesting that you do not care what others think or that you are too lazy to make the effort to dress better.

Where can I buy professional clothing without spending a fortune?

Shop at outlet malls and check department stores (like Macy's) for sales. Other options are Nordstrom Rack, TJ Maxx, and Ann Taylor Loft.

Why are corporate casual dress codes being eliminated in many settings?

The informality of these dress codes gave many people the impression that there were no guidelines or boundaries between dressing for work and relaxing at home. This had a negative impact on professional image and work ethic.

How do I know if my body language is detracting from my professional image?

Ask a colleague for feedback. Videotape yourself.

Is it acceptable for men to wear baseball caps inside?

No. It is considered bad manners. Hats should be removed when entering a business or room.

 Do you have any tips for men wearing suspenders?

Suspenders should be matched to the tie. A subdued or flashy pattern should be compatible with the company culture.

 What about tattoos?

Keep them hidden. Don't get tattoos on your hands or face. The tattoo becomes part of your image and may hurt your chance of getting a job or getting promoted.

 Is it professional for men or women to wear cologne or perfume in the work setting?

Subtlety is the key. Remember, you are not an air freshener. Moderation is best. If people comment about your scent in the afternoon, you are using too much. Also, if your scent lingers in a room after you've left, you are using too much. Be sensitive to the fact that many people are allergic to cologne and perfume.

TAKE-AWAY TIPS

✓ You will have a better chance of feeling good on the inside if you look good on the outside.

✓ Dress for the job you aspire to, not for the job you have.

✓ Wear clothes that fit well. Invest in a good tailor or seamstress.

✓ Your clothes affect your credibility.

✓ Don't wear sunglasses inside.

✓ Sloppy clothing may imply sloppy work.

✓ How you present yourself is how most will know you.

✓ Unfortunately, the words you say can be undone by your body language.

4

Interviewing

What You Say Gets You What You Want

Do you:

Know what to expect during an interview?
Know what to wear during an interview?
Know what to bring to an interview?
Know what to do if the interviewer asks you a question you can't answer?
Know how to react to the unexpected during an interview?

Are you:

Nervous before and during an interview?
A less-than-stellar interviewee?

These are legitimate concerns that can add to the normal stress of an interview. The trick is to know how to prepare and present yourself so you can minimize anxiety and maximize your level of confidence. This chapter provides guidelines to support you in any interview or even any business meeting.

Preparing for the Interview

What should I do before the interview?

Find out as much as you can about the company (for example, financial or Magnet status) or position. Check the website for information about the people in charge. For example, if you are interviewing with a manager who wrote an article on civility, you could mention the article during your interview. The more you find out, the more prepared you will be and feel.

You also need to review your public persona. Make sure your information presents a professional and positive impression. Prospective employers often search the Web for information on you and may locate your website, blog, or social networking profile (LinkedIn or Facebook, for example). You should be able to substantiate anything you post online about degrees, professional accomplishments, awards, military service, job titles, length of employment, and so on. Make sure you have nothing there (words or pictures) that could embarrass you or your potential employer.

Never trash anyone online. Keep your personal information personal. Don't post about any illness or how you dislike your current place of employment or nursing colleagues.

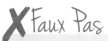 **X Faux Pas**

John did a great job promoting himself for a cardiovascular sales position in a pharmaceutical company. He eloquently described his various job positions related to cardiac nursing. Unfortunately, when asked about the company's new cardiac drug that had received FDA approval a few weeks earlier, he could not answer the question. One look at the company's website would have informed him of this drug's approval and helped him to prepare himself accordingly.

What should I do if there is something online that casts me in a negative light?

If possible, remove the negative item. LinkedIn and Facebook allow users to delete information. If you cannot remove it, be prepared to explain it—and that it is not a true reflection of who you are today. You could also add that you learned a valuable lesson about social media and regret that you cannot undo the picture or words.

Is it OK for me to request to connect with someone I interviewed with on LinkedIn?

No. I would not suggest this. You are not colleagues, nor are you in a situation to be of any benefit to the interviewer. If you are hired, you could reconsider this at a later date.

After the interview, can I ask to take a selfie with the interviewer?

No. The interview is not a social event. Don't trivialize it. It is a serious professional encounter with a potential job on the line.

Is it OK to post a selfie of myself in front of the medical center where I am interviewing?

No. Going for an interview is not like taking a vacation or going to an amusement park. Focus on getting the job.

Is it a good idea to have some names to drop?

Yes. Talk to family, friends, and people on the street, train, or bus. See if you can get a name to drop. Leverage those you know. When used appropriately, personal connections can

TIP

People like to do business with people they know and like. Responsible name-dropping can take you from the position of "stranger" to "insider" in the blink of an eye.

enable you to walk through a door opened wide rather than just get a foot in the door.

Try to familiarize yourself with names. If you are applying for a teaching position, learn the names of faculty members. Review their websites. If you can't pronounce a name, call the department secretary and ask. You can also get help online with pronunciation websites.

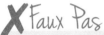

X Faux Pas

Peg received several long-distance calls on her answering machine from a hospital asking her for a reference. Because Peg was unaware of anyone interviewing who might use her for a reference, she did not return the calls. A week later, she ran into a former student who mentioned she had applied for an out-of-state job and had listed Peg as a reference. If the former student had contacted her sooner, Peg would have immediately returned the call to show her enthusiastic support of the applicant. The polite way to handle this situation is to ask permission before listing someone as a reference. Even if you have previously received a person's permission to use him or her as a reference, it is important to contact the person before any new job search to be sure nothing has changed.

If I have inside contacts, should I use them?

Yes. Talk to them before the interview about the position. What kind of personalities fit well in the job culture? What are the hidden expectations for employees? Why do people stay, and why do they leave? What is the turnover rate?

How can I find out who will be at the interview?

Call the person who scheduled you for the interview, explain that you want to be as prepared as possible, and ask if he or she can tell you who will be there. Find out the title of each interviewer and his or her role in the organization. This will help you direct questions to the appropriate person.

Often, you will be able to get biographical information on each interviewer on the organization's website. See if you have any commonalities. If so, bring them up during the interview. For example, perhaps you both went to the same college, did the same nursing internship, or served in the Army Nurse Corps.

What are some of the questions that may be asked?

The following list offers sample questions you might encounter. Role-play your response in less than 2 minutes. Write out your responses. Practice answering these questions out loud. Practice will help you sound more confident and avoid filler words and sounds such as *you know* and *um*. Be sure to allow time for spontaneous comments.

- What attracted you to the nursing profession?

- What experiences do you have that will help you in this position?

- What distinguishes you from other job candidates?

- What are your major strengths?

- What are your major weaknesses?

- Describe a difficult problem you faced in the past and how you resolved it. This is an example of a behaviorally based interview question. Also, questions could be centered around clinical scenarios. For example, if a patient has a BP of 90/60 and a HR of 130, what concerns might you have and what might you do?

- Tell me about a time when you learned to get along with a difficult person.

- Contrast a good decision with a poor decision you've made.

- How do you react to stressful situations?

- Where do you see yourself in 3 to 5 years?

- Have you ever worked with a group where you had to help people younger and less experienced than yourself?

- What experiences have you had working in teams?

Professionalism During the Interview

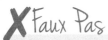

At the end of a job interview, Ryan asked the interviewer how best to follow up on the hiring decision. When the interviewer gave Ryan a phone number to call, Ryan asked if he could borrow a pen and piece of paper to write it down. The first thing the interviewer did once Ryan left was to make a note to himself: "Candidate was disorganized and did not even bring a pen and piece of paper."

What should I bring to the interview?

Bring a portfolio or folder with appropriate materials. For example, if you were asked to bring a professional license, make sure you have it in the folder. At the very least, bring the following:

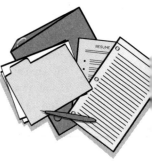

- A list of questions for the interviewer(s)

- A pad of paper or notebook for making notes or taking down follow-up information

- A writing utensil and a spare, in case the first gets lost or damaged

- Between 5 and 10 professional-looking copies of your resume

- Information about accessing your e-portfolio, if you have one

What should I wear to the interview?

Wear a dark suit unless you were advised to wear something else. Avoid yellow, red, or pink suits. However, these colors are fine for accessories or accent pieces. Stay away from long, dangling jewelry. Some human resource experts recommend the "rule of five" for jewelry. This limits jewelry to five pieces, such as two rings, a watch, earrings, and a necklace.

Make sure the suit fits well and all accessories match. Clothing is never neutral. It either adds to or detracts from your appearance.

Shoes are important, too. For men, leather soles are best. Before the week of your interview, try on the suit to make sure your shoes are the right height if you are wearing slacks. Give yourself time in case you need alterations in length or different shoes. Even if employees dress casually, job seekers are expected to dress more formally. This shows that you are taking the interview seriously and that you respect the company.

Make sure your hygiene is flawless. A wrinkled shirt, food caught in your teeth, or chipped fingernails can detract from your professional impression.

If you are commuting from your current job to attend an interview, you may not have time to change into professional clothing beforehand. Mention this to the hiring manager. Make sure he or she knows that you would have liked to have dressed more professionally but were unable. Managers may

✓ **Good Idea!**

Monica was finishing her junior year of college and applying for summer internships. She recently attended a seminar about business etiquette and thought she needed to purchase a suit for her interviews. Because her mother disagreed with her, Monica emailed the seminar speaker to specifically ask about the suit. The speaker supported Monica's position and reviewed the reasons for purchasing a suit. Monica felt confident and professional in her suit, did great during her interviews, and was offered the internship she wanted.

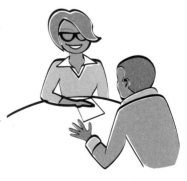

not care if they know your timing was tight and you did not want to call attention to the fact that you were interviewing for a position elsewhere.

Clothes are never a frivolity. They always mean something.

--James Laver

 Faux Pas

There was a buzz in the hallway outside one of the meeting rooms after a presentation. The female speaker had worn a white suit. Her red underwear could be seen through her suit, which distracted the audience from listening to her presentation. Her clothes undermined her professionalism and expertise.

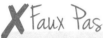 **Appearance and Hygiene Checklist**

Men:

Freshly bathed and shaven (even if interview is later in the day)

Clean fingernails

Deodorant applied

Teeth brushed

Clean, ironed clothes

Shoes polished

Minimal amount of cologne

Women:

Freshly bathed

Clean, manicured fingernails

Deodorant applied

No excessive jewelry, makeup, or perfume

Wearing a bra with no underwear showing

Clean, ironed clothes

Clothes that are not too tight, too sexy, or too short

Shoes polished

✗ Faux Pas

Mary had worked in a hospital and was used to wearing scrubs. When she interviewed with a pharmaceutical company, she thought wearing a sweater set would be fine. She was embarrassed when she saw that she was the only one not wearing a suit. It is always better for clothing to be more formal than too casual. This shows respect for the interviewer and demonstrates that you made the effort to present yourself in a professional manner.

You can't climb the ladder of success dressed in the costume of failure.

–Zig Ziglar

What about body piercings and tattoos?

A common stand on body art and piercings is, "We don't care what you have pierced or tattooed, as long as we don't see it." Limit any visible piercings to the earlobes and keep tattoos covered, if possible. Remove the jewelry item from piercings that cannot be covered (pierced tongue, eyebrow ring).

Is it OK to smoke while waiting for an interview?

Absolutely not. If you smoke, try not to do so before the interview. Otherwise, your clothing will reek of cigarette smoke—a definite turnoff for many people. Don't smoke anywhere inside or outside of the facility. Also, be aware that many healthcare facilities do not hire smokers. Tobacco use can be easily detected by a lab test.

How can I be sure I'm on time for the interview?

If possible, visit the interview location before the day of the interview to plan the best route to avoid potential traffic pitfalls. Find out where to park and note the entrance to the building. This will eliminate a major stress on the day of the interview.

Allow extra time for traffic and accidents on the day of the interview. Make sure you have all relevant phone numbers with you. If you get stuck in traffic, call your contact and notify him or her that you might be late. Tell the person you will call back with an update.

Always plan to arrive at least 30 minutes early. This will give you time to park, take care of personal business, and orient yourself to the medical center. Find out where your interview will be held. But don't report there until 5 or 10 minutes before your scheduled interview. In the interim, relax in the lobby or coffee shop. Bring a professional or other business-oriented magazine or book to read while waiting. This will demonstrate that you are serious about continuing to learn and improve professionally.

Allow time to use the restroom and check your appearance before presenting yourself to the receptionist 5 to 10 minutes ahead of time. Be sure to greet the receptionist with courtesy and respect. **Remember:** The receptionist may be asked by the interviewer to comment on your behavior and manners. Wait for the receptionist to advise you on where to sit.

Should I come prepared with some questions?

Yes. This shows careful preparation. If you don't have any questions, it may look as if you are either unprepared or uninterested. Here are two good questions to ask:

- What skills are considered most important for success in this position?

- What kind of educational opportunities do you offer to support career growth?

If all of your questions were answered, you could say something like, "My questions were all related to Magnet status and clinical ladders, and you covered them already."

Interview Dos and Don'ts

Do:

Use a firm handshake.

Wait to be offered a seat.

Have good eye contact with interviewer(s).

Maintain good posture.

Speak so you can be easily heard, but not too loudly.

Be direct and to the point without rambling.

Turn off your cell phone and any other electronic devices.

If you have an emergency situation and may need to be contacted, explain that at the very beginning of the interview.

Don't:

Use a limp or crushing handshake.

Chew gum.

Sit down until you are directed to do so.

Give one-word answers.

Give long, drawn-out answers.

Interrupt anyone who is speaking.

Bad-mouth a previous employer.

Order an alcoholic beverage if you are taken to lunch.

Comment about nationality, age, religion, or photographs of family or children.

During an interview, it is OK to ask when I can expect to hear about the position?

Yes. This is a reasonable question. You might say, "I am confident that I would do a good job. What is the next step in the selection process?" You can also ask about the timeframe for filling the position.

Things Not to Say in an Interview

"Do you have a smoking area?"

Smoking is a turnoff and may make you unemployable in healthcare. Medical insurance may be higher for smokers.

"I'm not sure what to do with my kids if I get this job."

This suggests you may have childcare problems.

"I really need this job to get away from my home situation."

This is too personal and could affect your ability to perform your job effectively.

"This city has great bars!"

Will you have a hangover on Monday?

"Are those pictures of your children?"

It is inappropriate to discuss children, regardless of whose children they are, in interviews. The conversation could lead into delicate or possibly illegal areas and may make the interviewer uncomfortable.

"Do you have disability insurance?"

The interviewer may wonder if you are trying to get a job to go on a disability claim. It is illegal to discriminate against anyone with disabilities.

Marianne P. Deska, human resources consultant (personal communication, 2007)

What if I am asked a question that is not legal?

Questions designed to obtain information about age, gender, race, religion, marital status, physical and/or mental status, country of origin, sexual preferences, and any other discriminatory factors are generally illegal for making employment decisions. If you are asked an illegal question during an interview, you have a few options:

- Answer truthfully if you think your answer will not hurt your employment potential.

- Inform the interviewer that the question is illegal, but be aware that by doing so, you run the risk of appearing confrontational or uncooperative.

- Examine the intent behind the question and respond with an answer related to the job. For example:

  - **Illegal question:** "Who is going to take care of your children when you work extended hours?"

  - **Possible answer:** "I can meet the work schedule that this job requires."

Table 4.2 includes examples of illegal and legal questions you may be asked in a job interview.

4.2   **Examples of Illegal and Legal Questions During a Job Interview**

Illegal	Legal
Are you a U.S. citizen?	Are you authorized to work in the U.S.?
How old are you?	Are you over the age of 18?
How many kids do you have?	Can you work overtime if needed?
What is your height and weight?	Can you lift a 50-pound weight and carry it 100 yards?

continues

4.2 Examples of Illegal and Legal Questions During a Job Interview *(continued)*

Illegal	Legal
Are you an alcoholic?	What was your attendance record at your previous job?
Do you go to church?	Can you work on Saturdays and Sundays?

What should I do if I don't get a positive response about the next step in the interview process?

Ask the interviewer if he or she has any areas of concern. Try to clarify any misunderstandings. Ask again about the next steps and the hiring timetable.

What should I do at the end of the interview?

Shake hands and thank the interviewer(s). Say goodbye to the receptionist. Remember his or her name. If someone walks you out, this is still part of the interview. Don't let your guard down and be careful of what you say.

Maintain professional behavior and manners as you exit and get into your car. Don't light up a cigarette or take off your jacket as you walk out of the building.

Top 10 Interview Blunders

1. **Making negative comments about former employers, supervisors, or co-workers.** No matter how bad they were, bashing them *never* makes you look good!

2. **Giving a call-back number that leads to an unprofessional outgoing voice-mail message or using an inappropriate email address.** Avoid loud music, toddlers attempting to say "Mommy/daddy isn't home," or slang on your voice mail. Be aware that your email address can reveal a lot about you. Avoid addresses like happygirl69@gmail.com. It's worth the extra effort to create a professional email address for job searches. Email accounts are free and easy to set up. This is discussed more in Chapter 7, "Avoiding Blunders with Social Media."

3. **Wearing inappropriate attire.** Flip-flops, plunging necklines, exposed thongs, sweatshirts, or spandex material of any kind is never appropriate. If you have to ask yourself or someone else, "Does this look OK?", then it most likely doesn't.

4. **Arriving too early or too late.** Arriving late obviously sends a bad message, but arriving more than 20 minutes early at the interview site can send a bad message as well. Simply put, it's annoying. Remember, it is good to arrive early at the medical center for your interview. This gives you plenty of time to park, take care of personal needs, and orient yourself to the center. But, don't present yourself too early for the actual interview. Five or ten minutes is appropriate.

5. **Divulging too much personal information.** No matter how much you want or need the position, do not dissolve into tears about your marriage woes or childcare issues. This will not help you get the job.

6. **Cell phone interruptions.** Even on vibrate only, a cell phone going off is still a distraction and potentially sends the signal that you will be taking too many personal phone calls. Always turn off your cell phone!

7. **Incomplete or incorrect contact information on your resume or application.** Take time to update former employer and reference information. Also, make sure it does not have any typos. Have someone else read your resume before you send it out.

8. **Inability to speak about or recognize past mistakes or weaknesses.** Everyone drops the ball sometime. Be prepared to talk about it and explain how you grew from the experience.

9. **Bringing friends, children, or significant others with you to an interview.** You'll be expected to perform your job without their support. Having them there will be unprofessional and can make you appear too eager and needy.

10. **Lack of enthusiasm.** This is especially bad for a new graduate. A winning attitude and desire to learn can easily make up for lack of practical experience. Make sure you get plenty of rest before your interview so your eyes are bright. Smile and show your enthusiasm.

Nicole Nardi, BSN, RN, former nurse recruiter
(personal communication, 2007)

After-Interview Professionalism

In a recent job interview, I was encouraged to follow up by email. Is this OK?

This is something new that is now acceptable in many settings. The advantage of this is that it allows for immediate follow-up and the ability to respond quickly to questions or concerns. It also keeps you in the manager's mind.

Should I write a thank-you note after the interview?

This form of etiquette is changing. Many hiring managers prefer getting an email within an hour or so after the interview. If you want to follow the email with a handwritten note, you can do that. Write clearly and neatly. If you type a note, limit it to two short paragraphs. It may be wise to ask the interviewer how he or she would prefer for you to follow up.

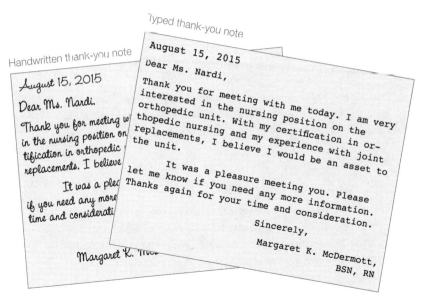

Typed thank-you note

August 15, 2015

Dear Ms. Nardi,

Thank you for meeting with me today. I am very interested in the nursing position on the orthopedic unit. With my certification in orthopedic nursing and my experience with joint replacements, I believe I would be an asset to the unit.

It was a pleasure meeting you. Please let me know if you need any more information. Thanks again for your time and consideration.

Sincerely,

Margaret K. McDermott, BSN, RN

Handwritten thank-you note

August 15, 2015

Dear Ms. Nardi,

Thank you for meeting w[ith me] in the nursing position on[...] tification in orthopedic [...] replacements. I believe[...]

It was a ple[asure...] if you need any more[...] time and considerati[on...]

Margaret K. [McDermott]

If I haven't heard about the position in the time anticipated, what should I do?

Call and say that you are "checking in" about the status of your application.

If I get a rejection letter or find out the position was filled, should I call and ask why I didn't get the position?

No. Send a letter or email saying that you know the position was filled and say that you are interested in other related positions. This keeps your name in the forefront and shows that you are not a sore loser.

Phone Interviews

I was hoping for a face-to-face interview and got scheduled for a phone interview. Is this a bad sign?

No. Often, phone interviews are a standard first step. They also minimize travel expenses for out-of-town applicants. In addition, Skype or other online video communication methods can be used for interviews.

What is the main purpose of a phone interview?

Phone interviews are a cost-effective, timesaving method for screening job candidates. As a job candidate, your goal is to determine if you are a fit for the organization. If so, your next goal is to get an invitation for an in-person interview.

How can I ensure a successful phone interview?

See the following list for guidelines to ensure a successful interview (Pagana, K. D., 2012a):

- **Prepare as you would for a personal interview:** Because there is no chance for eye contact or other nonverbal cues, you must be impeccably prepared. This is your only chance to make a good first impression.

- **Control your surroundings:** You must be able to talk freely without any distracting background noises. No crying kids or blaring televisions. Schedule the phone interview when you will be at your best and in total control of the situation.

- **Get into a business mode:** Many people dress professionally even for phone interviews because doing so causes them to feel and act more businesslike during the interview. If you are wearing pajamas, you may sound too casual or tired.

- **Stand up:** Your voice will sound more confident and dynamic. Move around a bit and use hand gestures.

- **Smile:** The smile on your face can be heard in your voice and projects a positive impression.

- **Have a pen and paper available:** Don't shuffle papers or waste time looking for something to write with. Take notes. Ask questions.

- **Don't give one word answers:** Rather than saying a simple *yes* or *no*, provide a short explanation.

- **Limit your answers to less than 2 minutes:** If the interviewer wants more details, he or she will ask.

- **Have your resume and supporting data in front of you:** You may be asked questions about your background and previous experiences. Be ready to answer them.

- **Don't interrupt the interviewer:** Be a good listener. You want to gather information to see if you are a good fit for the organization.

- **Turn off the call-waiting option on your phone:** The beep is distracting. Besides, you should not put the interviewer on hold to take another call.

- **Watch your manners:** Use the person's title and his or her last name. Don't chew gum, eat, drink, or smoke. It's OK to have water handy in case your mouth feels dry.

- **Close the interview:** Ask about the next step in the interview process.

- **Send a thank-you note after the interview:** As noted, this can be by email and/or regular mail.

Do you have any recommendations about outgoing voice-mail messages?

This could be your point of contact regarding the next step in the interview process. Make sure your voice-mail message reflects a professional persona. Although your friends may enjoy hearing a snippet of your favorite music, the interviewer may find it annoying and off-putting.

Frequently Asked Questions

 Should I ask permission before listing someone as a reference?

Yes. Ask the person if he or she is willing to serve as a reference. Then send the person a thank-you note and a copy of your resume so he or she will be up-to-date on your job situation. References may also be obtained via online forms. Make sure your references are on the lookout for these forms and that they fill them out quickly. Of course, you need to be certain you have the correct email address for your reference.

 What should I do with my coat?

Take it off before you get to the interview area. Fold it over your left arm so your right hand is free for shaking hands. Ask the receptionist where to hang it.

If there is candy on the table, is it OK to take a piece?

No. You want to be free to talk without food in your mouth.

May I bring a water bottle into the interview?

Only if you keep it in your purse or out of sight. Don't put anything on the interviewer's desk. If there is a table in front of you, you may put your interview folder on it.

What if I am asked a question that I cannot answer?

Think about it for a few seconds. Then, simply say, "I don't know," or "I can't answer that question." Don't apologize. If you know where or how to find the answer, you can explain that. This demonstrates your resourcefulness. You could also say, "I don't have an answer to that right now. Can I think about it and can we come back to it later?"

Is it OK to ask about salary in the first interview?

In general, no. It is better to focus on getting them interested in you and wanting you for the position. Save the salary question for subsequent interviews. However, if you are applying for a high-level position with wide variations in salary, this may be appropriate. You don't want to waste your time or their time if the salary range is not going to meet your requirements.

What if I am asked about salary?

Do your homework before the interview so you know what this type of position pays. Say you are looking for something in the salary range that is appropriate for the position.

What should I say when an interviewer asks about my major weakness?

Mention an area related to the job, but not required for the position for which you are applying. For example, suppose you are applying for a teaching position in medical-surgical nursing. You could say, "I have several ideas for articles, but I have not published anything yet. I am planning to attend a writing and publishing workshop later this year." Another example relates to a new graduate nurse without experience. He or she could mention prioritization as a weakness. This is something that would be expected, and thus not really a weakness. It is something that will be overcome with time.

 May I ask about advancement opportunities?

Yes, but be careful you don't give the impression you are too ambitious and are mentally planning your next career-advancement move.

 Is it OK to talk about interviewing with other companies?

Yes, but be careful. It might be better not to mention other companies until you are discussing salary or you are asked, as opposed to bringing it up yourself. Leveraging your situation with other interviews is a great way to make you seem more desirable. If the interviewer is worried about losing you to a competitor, your bargaining position can improve.

 How can I get correct names and titles of interviewer(s) for writing thank-you notes?

Ask for a business card, check the company's website, or call the office. If you call the office, say you are writing thank-you notes and want to be certain that you have correct names and titles.

 How should I prepare for a phone interview?

Prepare as thoroughly as you would for a regular interview. Your goal is to be invited for an in-person interview.

Will standing up during a phone interview make my voice sound more confident?

Yes. Try recording a message sitting and standing and you will see the difference.

Is it OK to post something on social media after my interview?

I would not do this. It is not professional. It may be a turnoff to a prospective hiring manager if he or she reads your thoughts regarding the interview process.

TAKE-AWAY TIPS

✓ Grandma's right: You never get a second chance to make a good first impression.

✓ Dress for the role to which you aspire.

✓ Turn your cell phone off before your interview. If it goes off by mistake, apologize and quickly turn it off without answering it.

✓ Never bad-mouth former employers during the interview.

✓ Answer the employer's questions in 20 seconds to 2 minutes.

✓ You can increase your chances of getting a job by projecting a positive, upbeat, confident, and mature attitude during interviews.

✓ Ask the interviewer for a business card. This will give you the correct spelling of his or her name, his or her title, and the address for writing a thank-you note.

✓ A smile on your face during a phone interview can be detected in your voice.

✓ Sending a thank-you note or email demonstrates good people skills.

5

Meetings Still Matter

Making Meetings Work for You

Do you:

Think meetings are important in the current climate of change?

Wonder if you need to schedule a meeting?

Consider meetings a waste of time?

Know how to run a productive meeting?

Know the responsibilities of a meeting's leader and participants?

Wonder about the seating arrangements?

Meetings are still a vital aspect of most businesses. They provide opportunities to distribute information, strengthen team-building, support business relationships, and display leadership potential. In addition, they enable members to take measure and evaluate each other. Some meetings, however, are unnecessary, boring, and unproductive time wasters. These negative components can be avoided when meetings are well-planned and properly conducted.

Planning and Preparation

What is the first step in planning a meeting?

The first step is to determine the purpose, goal, or outcome of the meeting. This will help guide the meeting's who, what, when, where, and why.

If, for example, the purpose of the meeting is to discuss a new healthcare requirement, you should provide that information ahead of time so discussion can take place at the meeting. If your purpose is to generate ideas and brainstorm, you must actively encourage participation.

How do I know how much time is needed for the meeting?

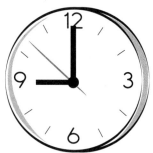

Timing is important. You must consider the purpose of the meeting along with the time constraints of the participants. Don't waste people's time. Most meetings should not exceed one hour.

When scheduling a meeting, are there time slots to avoid?

It is usually best to avoid scheduling a meeting early or late in the day, Monday morning, Friday afternoon, religious holidays, or the afternoon before a holiday. People are often busy, unavailable, or simply distracted at these times.

Can I use technology to help set up a meeting?

Yes. Outlook, Google Calendar, and Doodle can all be used for scheduling meetings. Meeting set up using these types of programs will appear on a person's work calendar.

You may even have the option of checking the schedules of other meeting participants prior to sending out an invite. However, not all schedules will be up-to-date. Sometimes, it may be best to send out an email with potential dates and times before scheduling.

How do I determine the location for a meeting?

This depends upon the degree of formality or informality necessary for the purpose of the meeting. The meeting could be housed in a boardroom or in the cafeteria. Things going on outside the room should not distract participants. If possible, the location should be convenient for the majority of the participants.

The setting should be accessible and appropriate to those with disabilities. People with visual impairments or hearing difficulties should sit near the speaker. Wheelchair access should be considered if needed.

What should be included in the agenda?

This will depend on the type of meeting. An informal meeting may have only a few topics for discussion. An agenda for a more formal meeting usually includes the following:

- Date and location
- Start and end time
- Topics to be discussed, with the responsible person listed and time allotment
- If the meeting is scheduled near a mealtime, note in the agenda whether food and drinks will be provided.

What is the typical order for items of business on a committee meeting agenda?

The typical order is usually as follows:

1. Welcome and call to order

2. Approval of the minutes from the last meeting

3. Reports

4. Old business

5. New business

6. Announcements

7. Adjournment

If you are new to the chairperson role, use previous meeting agendas as a guide.

Reasons to *Not* Have a Meeting

How do I know when to *not* have a meeting?

Unfortunately, many meetings are held that should not have been scheduled. Before planning, determine whether the meeting is really necessary. Here are some reasons to *not* have a meeting:

- **You are planning to rubber-stamp a decision you have already made:** If you have no intention of listening to the suggestions and opinions of others, don't waste their time at a meeting.

- **Your goals can be accomplished through email:** Consider whether people really need to be physically present at a meeting. Is it worth the time and energy to get people away from work for a meeting?

- **You want to communicate a message to one member by avoiding an uncomfortable one-to-one discussion:** Don't use meetings to camouflage your motives and responsibilities.

- **Your agenda is not clearly defined:** This can result in a rambling, unfocused, and long meeting.

- **You just want an audience to hear yourself talk:** This wastes people's time. Committee members will probably zone out and may avoid future meetings that could be important.

What options do I have if asked to attend a meeting that is usually unproductive?

Here are some ways to imply that you do not want your time wasted:

- Ask whether your attendance is mandatory or optional.

- Ask whether you can send a representative in your place.

- Ask whether you can offer input by phone or email.

- Say you are unavailable, and ask whether the meeting is important enough to change your schedule.

People who enjoy meetings should not be in charge of anything.

--Thomas Sowell

Chairperson Etiquette

How should the chairperson run the meeting to ensure it is a good one?

The biggest mistake the chairperson can make is to assume that a well-planned meeting will run itself. Here are some important guidelines for running a good meeting:

- Distribute the agenda by email before the meeting.

- Attach supporting materials (including minutes for approval) to the agenda. Sometimes, this material is posted online at a secure site to ensure privacy.

- Request confirmation of attendance. This can be done electronically.

- Arrive early to greet participants.

- Inform participants of the seating arrangements.

- Start and end on time.

- Follow the approved agenda.

- Speak in a voice that is easily heard.

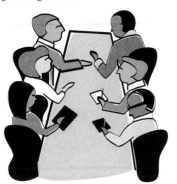

- Use professional visual aids.

- Keep control of the meeting.

- Schedule breaks if needed.

- Don't recap information for latecomers.

- Use effective facilitation skills so participants can ask questions and express their views.

Helpful Tips for Facilitating Meetings

- Set the tone for the meeting at the beginning.
- Clearly state the purpose of the meeting.
- Use double-sided place cards on the table to learn names.
- If a certain person at the meeting has the specific information you need, pose the question directly to that person. This is more efficient and direct.
- Don't shy away from sensitive subjects.
- Keep the meeting on track. Don't let someone be long-winded or off topic.
- Summarize so everyone takes away the same message.
- Remember that the facilitator is not the focal point of the meeting. The facilitator draws others out.

(Adubato, 2005)

How can I prevent disruptive emailing and texting during meetings?

Convey your expectations early in the meeting. Remind people to silence or turn off mobile devices. Announce when you will be having a break so participants will know when they can check messages.

How do I keep meetings on track?

If a meeting starts to go astray, be polite and direct. Say something like, "That's a good point, and I'd like to discuss this with you after the meeting. Let's get back on track...." Another option is to redirect the conversation by asking a question. For example, "Now that we understand

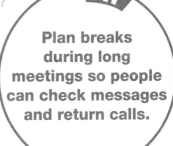

TIP

Plan breaks during long meetings so people can check messages and return calls.

the potential problems, what should be our next step?" If someone continues to filibuster, say something like, "Sarah, we understand your concerns. Let's hear from someone else."

✗ Faux Pas

A group of medical doctors was invited by the hospital CEO to attend a 1-hour meeting at 7:00 a.m. to share ideas for improving the healthcare system. A week before the meeting, the doctors received a folder of documents related to the system. On the scheduled meeting date, the CEO arrived 10 minutes late and spent the next hour reviewing the materials in the folders. Finally, at 8:10 a.m., the doctors were given an opportunity to provide input. However, because the doctors had scheduled office appointments with patients, they left the meeting feeling that their time and effort had been wasted.

How do I handle people who keep interrupting others?

As the chairperson, you must stop this behavior. Try saying one of the following:

- "Can we please hold that thought until later?"

- "John is getting to that point. Please let him finish."

- "Please let me finish."

Or, raise your hand to the interrupter and continue speaking.

TIP

A good leader shows respect for people's time.

What if the meeting ends early?

People will be delighted! Don't drag on to fill the time.

What if the meeting starts to run long?

Don't try to cram in the agenda. Prioritize and determine what to discuss. Schedule another meeting to complete the unfinished business.

Should I conduct an evaluation after the meeting?

Yes. This is important because how you run a meeting is a reflection of your leadership ability and style. If you evaluate the meeting while the particulars are still fresh in your memory, you can make improvements.

Here are some questions to ask yourself:

- Did you accomplish your goals?
- Did you invite the right people?
- Did any unanticipated problems crop up?
- Did you run out of time?
- Did you maintain control?
- Do you need to debrief with a supervisor or close colleague about the meeting?

TIP

Make sure you accomplish your must-dos before key people begin to leave.

If you are not satisfied with any of your answers, decide what corrective action you should take for the next meeting.

Sometimes, the chairperson will provide an evaluation survey for participants to complete. This can be done on paper at the end of the meeting or electronically afterward. Use feedback to make the meeting more productive and efficient.

X Faux Pas

A committee meeting was set for 4:00 p.m., and several participants arrived early. Unfortunately, rather than starting the meeting on time, the chairperson spent the first 10 minutes chatting about his recent trip to Paris. As a result, the meeting ran over. Not surprisingly, in their meeting evaluations, several committee members criticized the chairperson for not starting the meeting on time, accusing him of "grandstanding."

Etiquette for Participants

What are some etiquette guidelines for participants?

Your active participation is essential for the success of the meeting. Remember, you are there because someone thought you have something to contribute. Here are some key guidelines (Chaney & Martin, 2007):

- Respond to the meeting notice concerning your attendance.

- Punctuality is expected. Arrive between 3 and 5 minutes early.

- Introduce yourself to those you don't know and shake hands.

- Bring needed materials and the agenda. (Many people bring mobile devices containing all of the necessary information.)

- Come prepared to discuss items on the agenda.

- Bring a pen and paper for taking notes and following up.

- Watch your posture and body language. Be professional.

- Pay attention to the chairperson and other members.

- Stay for the entire meeting unless you have informed the chairperson in advance that you need to leave at a certain time.

What are some distracting behaviors to avoid?

Avoiding distracting behaviors is important. Remember, others in the meeting will be making judgments about and forming impressions of you. Here are some behaviors to avoid:

- Failing to read supporting material before the meeting

- Rolling your eyes and looking at your watch

- Doodling, playing with pens, chewing gum, or tapping your feet

- Reading mail or checking your mobile device

- Interrupting others or dominating the discussion

- Propping your feet up on an empty chair

- Falling asleep

- Not contributing to the discussion

- Putting yourself down by saying things like, "It's only my opinion…"

- Asking permission before making your point

Does it matter what I wear?

Yes. As mentioned, people will be judging you and forming impressions about you during the meeting. Dress professionally and demonstrate impeccable grooming.

✗ Faux Pas

Darby was a new nurse manager in the health system. The dress code for managers was a white lab coat over scrubs or other professional attire. One afternoon, all the managers received a request to meet with the CNO at 3:00 p.m. to discuss patient satisfaction scores. Unfortunately, Darby forgot her lab coat that morning and was embarrassed to be the only manager not following the dress code. She learned to always keep a clean lab coat in her office.

Is it OK to arrive for a meeting too early?

No. Arriving more than 10 minutes before the meeting starts can create an awkward situation. Those in charge may be ironing out last-minute details. If you arrive early and see that people are busy with last-minute preparations, step outside the room and wait until the scheduled meeting time.

What should I do if I know I will be late for a meeting?

Tell the chairperson that you will be late. With advance notice, the chairperson may be able to seat you in a place less likely to distract others. When entering late, walk in as unobtrusively as possible. While taking your seat, don't greet others, rattle papers, or get refreshments.

What should I do if I need to leave a meeting early?

Notify the chairperson ahead of time. Sit near the door so you will be less disruptive when leaving. Similarly, if you anticipate that a meeting may run late and you need to leave at the normal end time, explain your conflict before the meeting and sit by the door. On the other hand, if you don't need to leave early, keep the seats near the door open for those who do.

What if I think I should have been invited to a meeting, but was not?

You can interpret this in one of several ways:

- The organizer may have thought that your time would be better spent doing something else.

- The purpose of the meeting may be to make decisions above your level.

- The organizer may have made a mistake.

If you feel comfortable doing so, you can ask why you were not invited. If a mistake was made, it can be easily corrected.

How do I handle back-to-back meetings?

The best way to handle back-to-back meetings is to prevent them from happening in the first place. If possible, keep a 15 to 20 minute buffer zone between meetings. Also, be sure to allow for travel time. If you do have back-to-back meetings, it is a good idea to inform the chairperson before the meeting starts that you are on a tight schedule and will need to leave when the meeting is scheduled to end (Post, 2014).

Introductions and Seating

What is the proper etiquette for handling introductions?

The chairperson should arrive first to welcome participants and introduce new attendees. Another option is to have participants introduce themselves at the start of the meeting.

If an unknown guest is present, the chairperson should introduce that person at the beginning of the meeting and describe his or her role. Otherwise, people may be intimidated or distracted, trying to figure out why the person is at the meeting. If you don't explain why the person is there, they may think the worst—for example, that the person is there to discuss layoffs or cutbacks.

Meeting participants can also demonstrate initiative by arriving a few minutes early and introducing themselves to others. This is a great networking opportunity.

Where should I sit at a meeting?

If there are place cards, the answer to this question is simple. If not, it is polite to ask the chairperson where you should sit. Of course, you do not want to sit where the chairperson should sit. Avoid the head or foot of the conference table.

Where should the chairperson sit?

The person in the position of authority usually sits at the head of a rectangular table, farthest from the door. This is commonly referred to as the *power perch*. The seat to the right of the chairperson is usually reserved for his or her assistant or for the person next in importance. The person next in line of importance after that usually sits to the left of the chairperson (Chaney & Martin, 2007).

Because the chairperson usually arrives first to the meeting, he or she can sit anywhere in the room. Some chairpersons choose a seat that offers the best view of the room and enables them to engage the participants.

✘ Faux Pas

Marlene was delighted to be asked to join the Quality & Safety Committee. The meeting was held in the hospital auditorium at a U-shaped table in front of a projection screen. Marlene arrived early at her first meeting and took the seat in the center of the front table. She did this every month until one day she arrived a few minutes late and found the chairperson sitting where she normally sat. She was embarrassed to realize that she had been sitting in the chairperson's place every month.

Should place cards be used?

Using place cards is a great idea. It helps participants learn the names of others in the meeting. Two-sided cards are best. They enable participants to easily find their place, and to learn others' names.

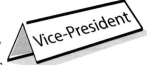

What if there are no chairs?

Conducting a meeting with no chairs, where everyone stands, works only if the meeting is short. In this case, you should minimize chit-chat and focus everyone on the task at hand. This would work for a clinical huddle.

Follow-Up Actions

What are the responsibilities of the chairperson after the meeting?

For the sake of proper etiquette, the chairperson should ensure that the meeting room is left in good order. Remove any plates, cups, papers, and trash from the table. The chairperson should also send a reminder to all participants indicating deadlines for completing follow-up tasks. Finally, the chairperson should arrange for the preparation and distribution of the minutes.

What are the main components of the meeting minutes?

The components of the meeting minutes differ by organization or committee. To gauge the amount of detail required, follow the format used by the organization or committee. In general, minutes include any or all of the following:

- The name of the group, the date, the place, and the time

- A list of participants (present, excused, and absent)

- Approval of minutes from previous meeting (with or without corrections)

- Reports from committees or officers

- Unfinished business and action taken

- Action taken on motions (who introduced and who seconded)

- Follow-up responsibilities

- The date and location of the next meeting

- The time of adjournment

- In some situations, notices protecting the confidentiality of the information

Serving Food and Refreshments

Are table manners important for meetings that include a meal?

Yes. Watch your table manners. You will be scrutinized, and your table manners will leave a positive or negative impression. You will feel more confident and comfortable if you follow proper dining etiquette. (See Chapter 9, "How Dining Etiquette and Business Success Go Hand in Hand")

Which meal is usually best for a business meeting?

Lunch is the most popular for the following reasons:

- It occurs during the workday and not on personal time.

- Providing food can motivate people to attend the meeting.

- It is short and time-limited because people have to get back to work.

- Whether significant others should be invited is not a concern, as it is with an evening meal.

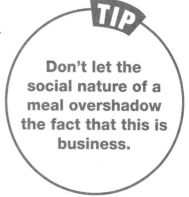

TIP

Don't let the social nature of a meal overshadow the fact that this is business.

What is the proper etiquette for handling the food and still participating in a business meeting in a professional manner?

Be polite and arrive early to get your food and drinks before the meeting starts. Avoid eating anything messy. If you should arrive late, don't distract others while getting food. Remember, you are there for business. Food is not the main priority.

See the following tips for etiquette during a breakfast meeting (Gould, 2014):

- If eating a croissant, break off a bite-sized piece and, optionally, add jelly or jam before eating it.

- Use a fork and knife to handle a gooey cinnamon roll. (Don't even think of licking your fingers!)

- Break muffins in half, and then break off bite-sized pieces. Butter each piece and then eat it.

- Butter and add jam to toast while it is on your bread plate. Cut the toast in half or quarters and eat each piece.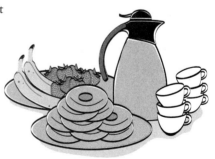

- Tear off a bite-sized piece of a doughnut and eat it. Only dunk it in coffee or tea in the privacy of your home.

If a meeting takes place in a restaurant, who pays the bill?

The person who scheduled the meeting pays the bill and tip. Note that this is regardless of gender.

Virtual Meetings

Why are virtual meetings popular?

Face-to-face meetings are costly in terms of travel and in terms of the human wear and tear that accompanies travel. Many companies have branches across the country or the world. Virtual meetings can connect people by computers, satellites, and phones. Examples include web conferences, WebEx, GoToMeeting, teleconferences, and videoconferences.

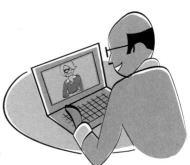

What are the advantages of virtual meetings?

In addition to saving time and money for travel, a key advantage is that participants can share information, discuss options, and make decisions in the privacy of their own offices without being distracted. Other benefits include the following:

- Scheduling is easier because participants are more flexible when travel is not involved.

- Real-time communication can take place between people in multiple locations and time zones.

- People are less likely to cancel because of personal issues because they can handle personal issues better in their home or office and still participate in the meeting.

- Participants can take turns presenting information without standing up, walking to the front of the room, and connecting their laptops to a projector.

- Large meetings can split into smaller sessions without the need for additional conference rooms.

- Some forms of web conference software generate full-text chat transcripts and audio recordings, enabling participants to review them later. This is also beneficial for those unable to attend the meeting.

- People won't come back to work exhausted and bleary-eyed after a red-eye flight from California to New York.

✗ Faux Pas

Edward was asked to participate in a conference call to discuss his proposal for a possible keynote during nurse's week. While traveling, he called in, only to find that the password he had been provided was incorrect. He tried calling the coordinator, but could not get through. Because he was out of his office, the meeting coordinator was unable to contact him—although she did leave a message on his office voice mail. When he finally thought to call his office 25 minutes later, he got the message, and joined the conference call late. Although this problem was not his fault, it did not provide a good first impression. To prevent this problem in the future, Edward now always obtains the cell-phone number of at least one person who will be at the meeting.

What are the disadvantages of virtual meetings?

The main disadvantage of conference calls is the absence of nonverbal communication, such as facial expressions, gestures, nods and other forms of body language. (Video calls allow some nonverbal communication.) Other disadvantages of virtual meetings include the following:

TIP

Make sure effective communication isn't being traded or ignored for bottom-line savings.

- Decreased opportunity for team building

- Decreased ability to control conversations that go on tangents

- Decreased spontaneity

- Potential for compromised confidentiality

- Potential for equipment failure

What is the etiquette for participating in virtual meetings?

Participant preparation is key to successful virtual meetings. Of course, participants also need to follow the meeting guidelines, reply promptly to messages, and protect confidential information. If videoconferencing is used, participants should remember to dress professionally.

TIP

Prior planning prevents poor performance.

Here are a few more tips (Schindler, 2008):

- Be polite.

- Log on at a specific time (often 10 to 15 minutes) before the meeting starts to test connectivity. Some online products require installation and download. If it is your first time participating in a virtual meeting, you may want to test the connection as soon as you receive the invite. That would give you more time to resolve any technical issues.

- Minimize background noise.

- Identify yourself before speaking every time.

- Avoid multitasking. Participate fully.

- Turn off all mobile devices.

What are some tips for planning virtual meetings?

The guidelines discussed earlier in this chapter for planning face-to-face meetings apply. Here are some important guidelines specific to virtual meetings (Post 2014; Schindler, 2008):

- Be alert to time zone differences. Timing and notifications are critical.

- Confirm availability of all invited participants.

- Send needed materials and make sure they have been received.

- Provide ground rules, such as when to use the mute button.

- Check equipment in advance.

- Make sure you are comfortable with the equipment or have a support person available. You can't run a good meeting if you are worried about which button to press.

- Determine a backup plan in case of equipment failure. Will you postpone the meeting or use backup technology?

- If you are participating in a videoconference, pay attention to your dress and body language.

> **TIP**
>
> Use a co-facilitator to handle the technology and have someone else take minutes while you run a virtual meeting.

What considerations should I make when participants live in different time zones?

Be aware of the participants' working hours. Consider how the meeting time will affect their work schedules—for example, requiring them to arrive extra early, cutting into the lunch hour, or keeping them late at work (Schindler, 2008). If the time is not good for some participants, rotate the time slot for the next meeting to make inconveniences more equitable. Try to be fair to all.

Should I use the mute button during a meeting?

People disagree about the use of the mute button. Those that like the mute button say it reduces background noise and improves sound quality. Those who dislike it often feel that meetings are more spontaneous and productive if people don't use the mute button. This sets the expectation for interaction. Not using the mute button also gives facilitators a better sense of each participant's level of engagement. With regard to the mute button, follow the instructions of the meeting chairperson.

How can I encourage participation during virtual meetings?

Here are several suggestions:

- Conduct a quick roll call at the beginning of the meeting. If a new person joins the call later, ask for his or her name at a good stopping point.

- Solicit audience feedback with polling features.

- Provide opportunities for each participant to speak without interruption for 30 seconds. Tell participants that if they wish, they can pass when their name is called. Another round of speaking opportunities later in the meeting may give those who did not speak the first time another chance to be heard.

- Direct questions to participants by name.

- Limit the size of the meeting. The smaller the number, the easier it will be for people to participate and be understood.

- Keep the meeting short to ensure engagement.

Is it OK to put my phone on hold during a teleconference?

Be careful about doing this. If using a company phone, an info-mercial or canned music may play while the phone is on hold. This would be disruptive and annoying.

How do I handle meetings with a mixture of in-room attendees and remote attendees?

It is a challenge for moderators to meet the needs of both audiences. This is tricky because remote attendees at conference calls cannot see the nods of heads around the table or the pause as people look through papers. They also can't hear low-volume conversations.

Moderators must provide an audible connection to remote attendees. They also need to direct their commentary loudly toward the microphone, while also encouraging others to do the same (Schindler, 2008).

The chairperson should regularly check back with the remote members. Participants need to be reminded that the remote people may not be able to hear when the noise level goes up in the room.

TIP

If conducting virtual meetings with international participants, see Chapter 12, "Going Global," for etiquette tips.

Frequently Asked Questions

(?) How do I handle disruptions from mobile devices at meetings?

Remind people to turn them off before and during the meeting. If a person is using a mobile device during a meeting, try asking him or her a question.

If I attend regular meetings, is it best to sit in the same spot?

No. For team building and to prevent forming cliques, don't always sit near the same people.

 What is the recommended time for scheduling breaks during meetings?

Ideally, break after 60 minutes, but definitely after 90 minutes. People need breaks to clear their heads and stretch their legs. Also, by scheduling breaks, you encourage people not to use their mobile device during meetings. They can check messages and return calls.

 How long should the break be during a meeting?

A good average would be 10 to 15 minutes. However, if there are a large number of participants and the restrooms are not nearby, you may have to add some time.

 How can I get people back from a break on time?

Point to the clock in the room and tell people the exact time the meeting will resume. In the absence of a clock, tell people the time on your watch so they can adjust accordingly. Restart at the designated time.

 If my meeting is out of time and I need an additional 20 minutes, should I keep going and finish up?

No. You must respect people's time and other commitments. Often, people react to ending times as psychological breaking points. When the clock ticks over the allotted time, their minds begin to wander, they lose focus, and they may start feeling resentful. Only continue a meeting if doing so is agreeable to all attendees. Give people permission to leave if they need to.

If I am meeting to resolve a conflict, how do I determine a meeting place?

Aim for a neutral place that does not favor any of the participants. For example, rather than meeting in the CEO's office, meet in a conference room, which does not contain the CEO's diplomas and awards.

 What advice would you give for using technology with virtual meetings?

Use only the amount of technology needed to accomplish the desired meeting outcome. Keep it simple so you can focus on your message and not on the technology. Only use WebEx if a presentation is going to be done. If not, a conference call is all that is needed when the meeting is only going to entail conversation.

 How can my career benefit from participation in meetings?

Meetings provide you with an opportunity to network and to learn more about an organization. How you handle yourself can demonstrate your leadership potential.

 If I think the purpose of a meeting could be accomplished by email, should I say something?

Yes. I would contact the chairperson. He or she should appreciate the question and be able to make a final determination.

 If I have scheduled a meeting from 4 to 6 p.m., should I provide food?

Yes. This is polite because the meeting runs over a mealtime. Indicate on the invitation to the meeting what kind of food will be provided. For example, you may have hors d'oeuvres, light fare, or a full meal.

TAKE-AWAY TIPS

✓ Basic meeting etiquette applies regardless of location or whether the meeting is in-person or virtual.

✓ Watch your table manners if food is being served at a meeting.

✓ Before planning a meeting, determine whether it is really necessary.

✓ Active participation is key to the success of a meeting.

✓ If you have a reputation for starting meetings on time, people are more likely to arrive on time.

✓ When the business is done, the meeting should end.

✓ Don't allow a meeting to run over.

✓ For virtual meetings, place photos and short biographies of the meeting participants online or distribute the information with the agenda.

✓ Technology should support virtual meetings rather than drive them.

✓ Omitting the wrap-up of a meeting is like forgetting the closure of a speech. Include it in the time schedule.

✓ Airport lounges are a good option for meeting with out-of-town attendees.

✓ Multitasking is not conducive to an effective meeting.

6

Communication Technology

Controlling Technology Before It Controls You

Do you:

Know what to do if your cell phone rings during a meeting?

Want to demonstrate professionalism on a conference call?

Wonder if you should fax or mail a key document?

Know what should be included in an electronic signature?

Know what to do if your email system does not have a spell-check feature?

With today's technology, opportunity rarely knocks anymore. Instead, it presents itself in the form of a phone call, a voice mail, an email message, or a text message. Technology is fast, efficient, and inexpensive. As convenient and efficient as these forms of communication are, however, they can also be annoying, intrusive, and rude. It is easy to abuse communication devices (such as smartphones), text messaging, email, and instant messaging. This abuse can be costly to careers. If you want to present yourself in a courteous and professional manner, use etiquette with all forms of correspondence.

Politeness and consideration for others is like investing pennies and getting dollars back.

—Thomas Sowell

Email Etiquette

What are some tips for using email?

Email is now used more than any other type of communication. It is the primary form of communication in the workplace today. Whatever you write on email could come back to haunt you. Even deleted messages can be retrieved. Therefore, blunders become inerasable. Following are key tips to making email work *for* you instead of *against* you (Pagana, K. D., 2007b; Pagana, K. D., 2007c):

- **Never send confidential information via email:** Assume it will be shared. This information is one "forward" away from someone who may choose to use it against you or your company. Of course, anything patient-related is confidential. If you absolutely must send confidential information, mark it as such.

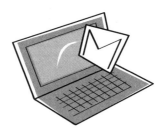

- **Make the subject line specific:** This helps the reader prioritize messages, file them, and easily retrieve them.

- **Include a greeting and a close:** It is more polite and less impersonal.

- **Use short paragraphs:** Being faced with an email with long paragraphs may cause the recipient to put off reading it. Three of four lines is good.

- **Never send long emails unless absolutely necessary:** These types of messages can be overwhelming. In the case of a long message, a phone call may be a better approach (unless you need to document something in writing).

- **Don't email if you're upset:** If you receive an email that elicits an emotional response, wait 24 hours before responding. Alternatively, pick up the phone and call the person to seek clarification.

- **Don't use all capital letters:** Doing so is considered the same as shouting.

- **Don't use all lowercase letters:** Doing so makes you look lazy.

- **Proofread before sending:** Use your email software's built-in grammar and spell-check tool.

- **Maintain a business-like tone:** Never use inappropriate language.

- **Check your recipients before sending:** This will avoid many errors.

- **Avoid overuse of the Reply All option:** Only include someone in your reply if absolutely necessary. Failure to do so annoys people and contributes to email overload.

- **Check your email regularly:** How regularly you check your email will depend on the type of work you do. But in most situations, you should plan to check it at least 2 or 3 times a day.

- **Occasionally check your spam mail folder:** That way, you can recover emails that were inappropriately tagged as spam.

- **Confirm your receipt of emails containing important information:** You can't assume the email got through unless you do this.

- **Respond to emails within 24 hours:** That is the general expectation of senders, who know you have more to do than answer emails all day.

- **When responding to a question, include the question in the response:** A message with just "yes" or "no" can be confusing.

- **Don't forward chain letters or anything else you would not want to receive:** This practice annoys people and adds to email overload.

TIP

Email provides a searchable record. You can be held accountable for things you send and receive.

X Faux Pas

A pharmaceutical representative was not happy with a secretary's help with his program setup at a hospital. After the program, he sent an angry email to the secretary that contained some foul language. The secretary forwarded it to the hospital president, who emailed the representative and permanently prohibited him from being on hospital grounds.

Should my email include a signature block?

Yes. The signature block should include your name, address, phone number, fax number, and email address. If you have an individual or company website, you could add the URL. If this is a business email, check to see if guidelines are available for font color and script. Your signature block provides several ways to contact you. Your address provides people with information necessary to identify your time zone, so they know when they can call you.

Setting up an email signature is very easy to do. For example, if you are using Microsoft Outlook 2013, go to the File tab and select Options. From there, select the Mail tab and click the Signatures button. Finally, type the signature you want to use and click OK. If you do not use Outlook, open your email program's Help feature and type *signature*, or ask your information technology (IT) support staff for assistance.

What is the recommended length of an email message?

Keep it short. Try to keep the entire message viewable without scrolling. Long messages can be tedious. Keeping messages short is especially helpful for people who check their messages on a mobile device. For long messages, it's better to simply call the recipient on the phone.

What should I do if my email program does not have a grammar and spell-check tool?

Copy the material and paste it into your word-processing program. Check the grammar and spelling there, and then copy and paste the text back into your email message.

Don't count on your spell-check program to catch everything. It may catch misspelled words, but it will not catch words that are spelled correctly but misused. (For more on these types of words, see Chapter 10, "Thank-You Notes and Business Letters.") It helps to read sentences backward to identify wrong words that are spelled correctly.

Is there an acceptable way to forward messages?

Forwarding is a great way to pass on material that may to beneficial to others, but be selective. Listed here are some forwarding tips:

- Forward only what your reader needs to see or reference relevant sections of the email chain.

- Don't forward confidential information or anything that is related to patients.

- Decide whether you should change the subject line.

- Eliminate the email header showing everyone who has received the message as well extraneous information, such as dates and times. Also remove any instances of the > symbol.

How can I remember to add an attachment?

Often, people intend to include an attachment, such as a word-processing document or image file, with their message, but forget to attach it. To avoid this, make it a habit to insert the attachment as soon as you mention it in the email. Do it before finishing your sentence or beginning the next one. This will prevent you from having to send a second email with an apology and the attachment.

If you are sending several attachments, find out if the recipient wants to receive them separately or all in one email. Multiple attachments may slow down the arrival of the recipient's incoming messages.

Depending on the size of the files, the attachments may need to be sent in multiple emails. If so, make sure the receiver is aware that several emails will be sent. Note in the subject or body the number of emails, for example, 1 of 5.

Is it best to cover one topic per email message?

Yes. This makes it easier for people to respond and easier to file the email. If this is not possible, number your items to simplify the response.

When should I use the BCC feature?

Use the blind carbon copy (BCC) when sending a message to multiple addresses. People do not like having their email addresses broadcast to everyone on your list. Put your name in the To box and the rest of the names in the BCC box. You should not give out someone's email address without permission.

It is not necessary to use the BCC when corresponding with a work team. These people know each other and probably already have other recipients' email addresses. In this case, put all of the addresses on the To box.

Is the BCC feature abused?

Yes. Be prudent with its use. When you use it, it is a clear indication that you are sending something behind someone's back. If you abuse this option, this can reflect poorly on you as someone who isn't forthright in dealing with co-workers or peers. Use it with caution. Also be aware that if someone in the BCC field uses the Reply All feature, the reply will go to everyone.

The ABCs of CCs and BCCs

If you're not sure when to use the CC and BCC features, follow these guidelines:

- **CC:** Use CC when you want someone to know something, and you want others to know that you want that person to know. This person does not usually need to respond.

- **BCC:** Use BCC when you want someone to know something, and you don't want others to know that you want that person to know (Shipley & Schwalbe, 2007)

Should I use an auto-responder or out-of-the-office assistant when I am unavailable?

This is a good idea when you will be unavailable for a period of time. People won't wonder if you received their emails. It will also tell them when you will return. The message should indicate whom to contact if immediate assistance is needed. (Note that some people choose not to do this for privacy reasons. They do not want people to know that they are away if they are on vacation.)

What things should I consider when setting up an email address?

Make sure it is professional. Here are some examples to avoid:

- mamabear@...

- sexymama@...

- billysmom@...

Cute or clever email addresses may be appropriate for personal messaging or social networking sites, but they are not appropriate for work. Use your full name whenever possible, and be sure to set up your email address display to show your full name on outgoing mail. If you don't know how to set up your email address in this way, go to the Help utility in your email software.

Are there situations when I should *not* use email?

Yes. Here are some examples:

- When resigning from a job.

- When sending a thank-you note for a gift.

- When discussing sensitive or confidential information, especially related to patients.

- When sending urgent information without follow-up. Computer glitches can happen.

- When you need an immediate response. Use the phone instead (Pagana, K. D., 2007c) or email and then call if you do not get an immediate response.

Do hospitals and other businesses have the right to monitor email?

Yes. The Electronic Communications Privacy Act (ECPA) upholds a company's right to monitor its email. This is based on the premise that the company provides and pays for the email; therefore, it owns it. It is best to not send personal emails from a work address.

Do you have suggestions for addressing email errors?

Because of the volume of email, errors are bound to occur. Worse, although email can get you in trouble, it typically doesn't get you out of trouble. Here are some helpful tips (Pagana, K. D., 2012b):

- Pick up the phone and apologize right away.

- Don't blame the mistake on email (for example, spell-check).

- Use the email recall function. Note, however, that this may make people more interested in reading the recalled mistake.

 Are there special guidelines for international email?

Yes. One is to be aware of differences in writing the date. Unlike people in the United States, who format the date as month/day/year, Europeans format the date as day/month/year, while people in Japan use the year/month/day format. So, for example, if someone in the United States types 5/6/15 in a message, it would mean May 6, 2015. In Europe, however, it would mean June 5, 2015. And in Japan, it would likely be interpreted as June 15, 2005. To avoid this problem, spell out the month, day, and year (May 6, 2015).

Telephone and Speakerphone Etiquette

How can I communicate my professionalism on the telephone?

The sound of your voice and your manners are essential components of phone etiquette. When speaking on the phone, smile, because the smile on your face will come through in your voice. Immediately identify yourself. Never assume someone will recognize your voice. Keep your full attention on the person with whom you are speaking. Here are some additional tips to follow:

- Keep background noise to a minimum.

- Concentrate on listening and avoid multitasking.

- Try to return calls within 24 hours.

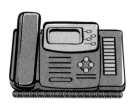

- Get organized before placing a call.

- Schedule phone conversations to avoid playing phone tag.

- Put callers on hold only when necessary. If you must put someone on hold, ask for permission.

- Don't answer your phone if you have a visitor in your office unless you are expecting an urgent call and have already informed your visitor of this possibility.

- Don't use call waiting in business situations.

- Avoid calling when you expect your contact to be busy.

- When returning someone's call, consider his or her time zone.

- Chewing gum on the phone is distracting.

- Be careful not to sneeze, blow your nose, or cough into the receiver.

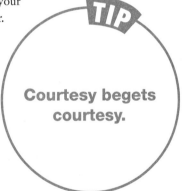

Courtesy begets courtesy.

What is the best way to transfer a call?

Always tell the caller the extension in case you are disconnected during the transfer. Brief the recipient about the caller so he or she can be prepared for the call.

What is the polite way to conclude a business phone call?

The person who initiated the call should bring it to a close. If not, the other person can politely ask if there is anything else to be settled. End on a positive note with a comment such as, "It's been nice talking to you," or "Thanks for your help with this project." Then, say goodbye and gently hang up the phone.

Do you have any suggestions for using speakerphones?

Yes. To avoid blunders, follow this advice:

- Always ask permission before putting someone on speakerphone.

- Ask if the person can hear you clearly. Many people find it hard to understand callers on speakerphones. You may need to turn up the volume.

- Close your office door when on speaker.

- Try not to rattle papers or make other noises that can distract the listener or make hearing difficult.

- Make sure you are not discussing patient information or other confidential data that can be overheard by those nearby.

- Don't use your speakerphone to listen to your voice mail. It is annoying to others who can hear it and could be embarrassing to the person who left a message intended only for your ears.

What can I do if I suspect someone has put me on a speakerphone?

If you are uncomfortable about being on speakerphone, say something like, "I'm having trouble hearing you. Would you please take me off your speakerphone?" Or, just ask if you are on speaker. The other person will usually pick up the handset (Pachter, 2013).

What is the proper etiquette for using caller identification?

You should use caller identification only to prepare for a call by identifying its source. It can create confusion and throw people off guard when they are greeted by name without having a chance to identify themselves.

✓ Good Idea!

After finishing graduate school, Matt was ready to interview for jobs in nursing administration. Before sending out resumes, he added a signature block to his email and updated his voice mail message to make it more professional. He got rid of the music that preceded his outgoing voice-mail message. He also Googled himself to make sure he would not be embarrassed by anything that an interviewer could find out about him on the Internet. (A growing number of hiring managers now search Google and social media sites for information on potential candidates before making a job offer.)

Cell-Phone Etiquette

How can I show respect for others and make myself a savvy cell-phone user?

Etiquette is about presenting yourself with polish and making those around you comfortable. It is hard to find an area in more need of consideration than that of cell-phone usage. See the following list for some strategies to make cell-phone usage professional (Pagana, K. D., 2009a):

- Don't let inappropriate ringing interfere with business. Turn off your phone.

- Don't answer a phone call while providing patient care and discuss another patient.

- Speak softly. Don't annoy or bother those around you.

- Turn your phone off or set it to vibrate at dinner meetings.

- Don't think you are so important that you need to be reachable every minute.

- Use your voice mail and return calls at an appropriate time.

- Make sure your voice-mail system is working and your mailbox is not full.

- Ask permission before taking someone's picture with your camera phone.

- Don't air dirty laundry in public. Keep a civil and pleasant tone.

How should I handle confidential information on a cell phone?

It is best to avoid discussing confidential information on a cell phone, especially if you are in a confined area with other people. People near you or the recipient may be able to hear your conversation. Be careful not to violate the privacy of another person by mentioning him or her by name or any other patient identifier.

What should I do if my cell phone rings during an interview?

Apologize and turn off your phone without looking to see who called. People have lost job offers because they answered their phones during an interview. Remember to turn off your phone before the interview.

X Faux Pas

A woman was in her final interview for a job position. She was the top candidate until her cell phone rang. She answered the call and proceeded to discuss her dinner plans. She was not offered the position.

Is it OK to put my cell phone on the table at an interview or in a restaurant?

No. It looks like you are expecting a call. Making or receiving a call on your mobile device is inconsiderate and intrusive in these situations.

Be a master of your phone, not a slave to it!

—Emily Post

What should I do if I need to be accessible by cell phone during a business meeting?

The vast majority of callers do not need immediate access to you. Of course, an exception would be if you are an expectant father or if you or a loved one is on a transplant list. In these cases and in other important circumstances, alert others prior to the meeting and keep your phone on vibrate. Excuse yourself and leave the room if you get a call.

What is the polite thing to do if I am talking on a cell phone and it is my turn to order at a service counter?

This has become a common problem. Get off your phone when it is your turn to order. For the sake of the attendant and those waiting behind you, focus only on your order. If you are in the middle of a call and your call is important, let the person behind you order before you while you finish your call.

Do you have any recommendations for talking while driving?

Many nurses drive to and from work. Talking on a cell phone while driving a car is dangerous. As a health professional, you don't want to end up in an emergency room. In some states, it is illegal to drive with a handheld cell phone. It has become such a big problem that police departments have begun including questions about cell phones in their accident reports. According to the National Safety Council, cell phones are now estimated to be involved in 26% of all motor vehicle accidents (2014). Driving performance, based on a cognitive distraction scale, is not much better using a hands-free device. Hands-free devices are dangerous because the driver is still distracted.

TIP

If talking on your cell phone in the car, let the person on the other end know if others are in the car and can hear the conversation.

Avoid using your phone in high-traffic areas or in tricky situations. Turn off your cell phone or let it ring. Check your voice mail when you get off the road. Pull off the road if you need to make a call while you are driving. Never read or send text messages while driving.

When Not to Use Your Cell Phone

Here is a short list. Basically, avoid using it anywhere you can bother or distract others.

- Worship services
- Weddings and funerals
- Public restrooms
- Libraries
- Doctors' offices
- Public performances and movie theaters
- Restaurants
- Meetings
- Public transportation

How can I use my cell phone in a polite manner at airports or train stations?

It is very important not to bother others, especially in enclosed areas where you trap those around you as unwilling listeners. Here are some suggestions (Pagana, K. D., 2009a):

- Speak softly and face away from others.

- Move away from close proximity to others.

- Speak briefly.

- Don't talk just to pass the time.

- Balance the convenience of the cell phone with the inconvenience it can cause others.

- Save any non-urgent calls for later.

Voice-Mail Etiquette

How can I make sure my voice-mail message conveys the right impression?

This is an important topic. Voice mail is a necessity for all professionals. How you use your voice mail can work for you or against you. See the following list for some guidelines to support a professional image (Pagana, K. D., 2011b):

- Jot down your key message points before you call.

- Always be prepared to leave a message. This will avoid *ahs* and *ums*.

- Be concise and brief. Show respect for the listener's time.

- Maintain a business tone. Don't respond when angry.

- Always state the purpose of your call. If calling patients, give them time to register who you are and what you are calling about.

- Don't say anything confidential in a voice mail. Others may overhear your message.

- Don't leave messages from noisy restaurants or parties.

- Be aware that voice mails can be forwarded to anyone.

- Don't play your voice-mail messages on a speakerphone.

- Don't use voice mail to avoid having a difficult conversation.

How can I avoid leaving a garbled message?

Enunciate clearly and speak slowly. Instead of saying "fifty," which can sound like "fifteen," say "five zero." Any number ending in "teen" can be confusing. State these numbers clearly, especially when mentioning drug dosages.

TIP: When you say your phone number, write it in the air or on a piece of paper. This will slow you down and give the person time to write it down.

If possible, listen to your message before sending it. Many voice-mail systems let you listen to your message, erase it, and start over. Take advantage of this functionality whenever possible. This is particularly relevant if you tend to pepper your messages with *ahs* or *ums*.

How can I sound confident when leaving a message?

Stand up and smile when you leave your message. Your voice will sound more confident if you are standing. Also, the listener will be able to hear the smile in your voice.

Is it appropriate to mention a good time for the person to call me back?

Yes, this helps avoid telephone tag. People appreciate this information.

If the person already has my phone number, should I leave it on a voice mail?

Yes. Leave your full name and phone number. This is more convenient for the person because he or she will not have to look it up. Say your name and phone number at the beginning and end of your message. Or, say them twice at the end, so the recipient does not need to replay your message.

How can I optimize my voice-mail message system?

Here are some tips to make sure your system is running well and will support a professional image (Pagana, K. D., 2007d; Pagana, K. D., 2011b):

- Check the outgoing message on your voice mail. Revise the greeting if it sounds unprofessional or if you hear distracting noises in the background.

- Test your system to make sure it is working. Having your phone ring indefinitely or having callers hear that your mailbox is full is unprofessional.

- Check your messages frequently so you can respond to all messages within 24 hours.

- Update your greeting message after a vacation or out-of-office period.

- Listen to all your messages before responding to any of them. A later message may negate the need to return a call.

Text Messaging Etiquette

Can texting affect your professional image?

Yes. Common courtesy is just as essential with texting as with other forms of communication. You need to be considerate and respectful.

Texting is about as informal as it gets. Some people send text messages routinely, while others may be unfamiliar with this method of communication. Ask professional people if they prefer to receive text messages over other methods of electronic communication. Older people may not check for text messages as often as younger workers. Therefore, texting can be challenging and unpredictable.

What are some guidelines for sending text messages?

You can't go wrong if you follow these tips (Pagana, K. D., 2012b):

- **Get to the point quickly:** No one wants to read a long message on a mobile device.

- **Don't text during meetings or presentations:** Doing so is rude. Others can see you clicking away or see the light from your screen.

- **Consider the time when texting:** Although you may be awake at 5:00 a.m., the sound of your incoming message may disturb a sleeping recipient.

- **Don't expect an immediate response to your text:** If the message is time sensitive, call instead.

- **Always check autocorrect:** Autocorrects are not always correct. They can be harmless, but they can also be inappropriate and hurt your reputation.

- **Proofread your message if using the voice-to-text feature:** Your phone can pick up background voices or noises.

- **Slow down:** Typing too quickly can result in errors. If a fast texting style suits your needs, proofread the text before you send it.

- **Never send bad news via a text message:** Call instead. The person may be upset and want to discuss the situation. This is especially important with patients.

How can I ensure that a text message won't bother me at night or at the movies?

Turn your phone off. Don't let your phone be your master. Be in control.

Is it possible to over-abbreviate in texting?

Yes. Abbreviations must be recognized to contribute to effective communication. Stick to company-wide abbreviations and avoid informal ones. If texting to patients, avoid abbreviations.

Fax Machine Courtesy

Is the fax machine dead?

Not yet. But its use has diminished markedly. However, it is still used a lot in healthcare. When sending or receiving a fax, HIPAA privacy requirements are an important consideration for patient information.

How can I extend courtesy to people on the receiving end of my fax transmissions?

A key consideration is to not send unsolicited faxes. Many people view them as worse than junk mail because they waste paper and tie up the machine. See the following list for some tips to guide you when you send faxes:

- Obtain permission before sending the fax.

- Always use a cover sheet and include the number of pages. This will alert the recipient if only a portion of the fax comes through.

- If the recipient uses a shared fax machine, call and let him or her know when you send a fax.

- If the message is more than a few pages, use another option for delivery, such as overnight or express mail.

- When composing a fax, use a slightly larger font so your message is easier to read.

- Consider the hour of the night or morning that a fax is sent, especially when dealing with a home office.

- Fax services such as FaxZero (www.faxzero.com) enable you to scan documents, upload them to a site, and then fax them to the receiver.

What should I include in a fax cover sheet?

The cover sheet should contain the name, address, phone number, and fax number of the sender and the recipient. It also needs the date, number of pages sent (including the cover sheet), and any pertinent messages. If delivery is urgent, that should be written on the cover sheet.

Frequently Asked Questions

? Is it OK to use emoticons in professional correspondence?

In general, these bouncy smiley faces are OK in personal emails, but don't use them too much in a business setting.

? Can I use just the subject line for a short email?

Yes. As an example, you could say, "Can we meet for lunch?" Then finish the sentence with "EOM," the acronym for "end of message" (Whitmore, 2005).

? Do you recommend using a signature line on a mobile device to excuse misspellings?

No. When you say, "Please excuse any typos because this was sent from a mobile device," it implies that you are unconcerned or in too much of a hurry to reread a message for mistakes.

? Does call waiting have a place in business?

Only use it if you are expecting an important call and you have told your current caller ahead of time. Otherwise, do not use it during a professional call. Using call waiting implies the unknown caller is more important than the person you are speaking with at the time. Ignore the clicks.

? Can people tell if I put them on my speakerphone?

Yes. The echo of a speakerphone is easily identifiable. You must ask permission before putting anyone on a speakerphone.

? What do you think of people who begin a phone conversation by saying, "How are you today?"

Don't begin your call this way. You will sound like a telemarketer. Start by identifying yourself.

If I called someone and we are disconnected, who is responsible for calling back?

You are. Because you placed the call, you know how to reach the person. The person may not know how to reach you.

 Is it OK to leave an important message on a voice-mail machine?

Yes. Only do so, however, if you follow up to make sure the message was received.

TAKE-AWAY TIPS

✓ Your email is a reflection of your professionalism or lack of it.

✓ Keep your personal emails out of the workplace.

✓ Smile when you use the phone.

✓ Schedule telephone appointments for important calls.

✓ Use speakerphones for conference calls only.

✓ Don't read or send a text message while driving your car.

✓ Ask permission before taking someone's picture with your camera phone.

7

Avoiding Blunders with Social Media

How Social Media Can Affect Your Career

Do you:

Google yourself and examine the results?

Think Facebook is a waste of time?

Have a LinkedIn profile?

Follow anybody on Twitter?

Know what kinds of photos are best for social media?

Know how a website is different from a blog?

The impact of social media has been demonstrated time and time again, from its role in political uprisings to its ability to influence decisions. As just one example of the power of social media, fans of actress Betty White on Facebook created a petition for White to host *Saturday Night Live*. Thanks to this petition, in 2010, White served as host on the popular show. Not surprisingly, because of its power, healthcare centers have made social media a key component of their marketing efforts to connect with patients.

Nurses have both obtained and lost jobs due to social media. One of the biggest concerns for nurses with regard to social media is maintaining patient privacy. This chapter will update you about these powerful communication tools and help you ensure that social media helps, rather than harms, you and your career.

Social Media Overview

Why do I need to know about social media?

Social media is changing the way people communicate. As with all new things, expect a learning curve. Whether you are texting, tweeting, blogging, or using Facebook, some etiquette guidelines apply. Learn to use these tools effectively and politely.

As a nurse, how can social media help my career?

Student nurses and nurses at all stages of their career can be helped by social media. Here are some of the key benefits:

- Learning things "hot off the press"
- Finding exciting jobs
- Getting help with your career
- Finding out about career fairs or educational offerings
- Networking with colleagues
- Meeting and connecting with new colleagues around the world
- Understanding professional dialogue
- Learning more about professional nursing issues

- Understanding many sides of a single issue

- Getting advice with clinical and professional dilemmas

- Answering questions and giving advice

Social Media Dos and Don'ts

Do:

Google your name and see what appears.

Evaluate your profile and postings.

Use your privacy settings to limit access to your information.

Be aware that what you post may affect your next promotion.

Be aware that private posts don't always stay private. Your information can be shared by others.

Tell your friends and colleagues not to post photos or videos of you without permission.

Post your accomplishments and interests.

Don't:

Post daily schedules, hotel room numbers, or home addresses.

Share too much personal information.

Post inappropriate photos or videos.

Trust all users on social networking sites.

Post anything you would not want a potential employer to read.

Criticize your manager or company.

Put people down, curse, or use racial statements.

Underestimate what people can learn about you on social media.

How can I be certain my social networking sites aren't harmful to my career?

Make sure your online information leaves no room for misinterpretation. Potential employers can view your profile. Many employers pre-screen applicants using social media. Inappropriate comments and photos can disqualify job candidates (Liburdi, 2008).

Employers will use social media tools to get to know you. They can use social media to learn about your contacts, how well connected you are, and your level of maturity. It pays to be aware of your public profile. Spend time building your online persona. See the box on the preceding page for some guidelines.

Do you have any guidelines for photos on social media?

Your profile photo—that is, the photo you use alongside your name on a social media site—will be part of the first impression you make on others. You do not want it to detract from your professionalism. For a professional site, like LinkedIn, use a professional photo. Photos help people know that they have connected with the right person. Here are some guidelines to help you (Pachter, 2013):

- Post a headshot.

- Make sure your face is in focus.

- Wear appropriate business attire.

- Choose a recent flattering photo.

- Consider hiring a professional photographer.

TIP

Be aware that if your profile photo is older than 10 years, people may be surprised when they meet you.

How much does it cost to use social media?

Most social media sites are free to use.

Can competency in the use of social media help me get a job?

Employers are looking for people who are proficient at social media. Digital trends affect every company, including healthcare. As an example, it would be hard to obtain a position as a nurse recruiter without this expertise. Competency in the use of social media can also help you keep your job. Blunders can result in job loss.

In some types of jobs, lack of competency in social media may raise a concern. This is especially true for baby boomers. Some companies may think people over 50 won't be able to use social media and other digital tools.

Complying with HIPAA on Social Media

Is it OK to discuss patients on social networks?

No. Nurses who do this may not realize that discussing patients on social networks can lead to a breach in confidentiality. Healthcare workers are subject to strict privacy and security rules. These were enacted in 1996 with the Health Insurance Portability and Accountability Act (HIPAA). This privacy rule went into effect in 2003 and set national standards to protect personal health information and medical records. The Security Rule, which took effect in 2005, set standards for protecting health information that is transferred in electronic form.

Can nurses violate regulations by sharing details about patients without mentioning the patient's name?

Yes. If, for example, a hospital employee has a casual conversation about a patient on the elevator, that could be a HIPAA violation. Nurses know it is ethically wrong to discuss this information in front of others. The challenge for healthcare providers is to realize that these same standards apply to online conversations.

X Faux Pas

Comedienne Joan Rivers passed away in 2014 after having a routine procedure at an endoscopy center. It was later reported that the personal doctor of the 81-year-old comedian snapped a selfie while Ms. Rivers was under anesthesia in the procedure room. This doctor also performed an unplanned biopsy on Ms. Rivers' vocal cords moments before Ms. Rivers went into cardiac arrest. The personal physician was not authorized to practice medicine at the private facility. The head of the clinic was let go. Legal ramifications will certainly follow (Otis, 2014).

What are some individual identifiers under the HIPAA Privacy Rule?

Although not an exhaustive list, the following are examples of identifiers (Pagana, K. D., 2011a):

- Names

- Photographs or images

- Social Security numbers

- Medical record numbers

- All elements of date (except year) directly related to an individual, such as birth date, admission date, discharge date, or date of death.

- Geographic subdivision smaller than a state

- Any unique identifying number, characteristic, or code

What are some of the legal ramifications for misuse of social media?

There are many serious consequences for nurses who use poor judgment on social media. Here are some examples (University Alliance, n. d.):

- Violations can be reported to the State Board of Nursing, resulting in reprimands, sanctions, fines, or the suspension of your nursing license.

- Violations of employment policies can result in penalties, including loss of job.

- Violations of state or federal law (such as HIPAA) can result in civil or criminal charges, fines, and possibly jail time. The healthcare facility or program affiliated with the nurse can also be subject to penalties and be named in a lawsuit.

Do professional nursing organizations have guidelines for using social media?

Yes. Take time to review the following:

- The American Nurses Association "Navigating the World of Social Media" (http://www.nursingworld.org/ FunctionalMenuCategories/AboutANA/Social-Media/Social-Networking-Principles-Toolkit/Fact-Sheet-Navigating-the-World-of-Social-Media.pdf)

- The National Council of State Boards of Nursing "White Paper: A Nurse's Guide to the Use of Social Media" (https:// www.ncsbn.org/Social_Media.pdf)

What responsibility do healthcare facilities have for social media use?

They need to inform employees about the risk of posting information on social media sites during and after work. Employers need to have clear policies for social media use inside and outside the workplace.

Here are some issues usually addressed in policies:

- Maintaining the organization's integrity, identity, and reputation ،

- Protecting patient privacy

- Using social media during work or on hospital property

- Not using your hospital email address as your primary means of identification

- Not expecting privacy for anything created, received, sent, or stored on the hospital computer system

- Being personally responsible for everything you post

- Understanding that violations are subject to disciplinary action, including job loss

Facebook

Why is Facebook so popular?

Facebook (www.facebook.com) enables users to stay connected and share information between friends. On Facebook, a *friend* is someone who has agreed to communicate with you and allow you some level of access to personal information. Members connect by issuing a *friend request*. You can also connect by letting Facebook search your email contacts or by looking at the lists of other friends' friends.

Nurses primarily use Facebook to connect with family and friends. With the exception of following professional groups, its use is primarily social and not work-related. Problems can result when work issues (such as patient concerns) spill over into social chatter.

What is usually part of a Facebook profile?

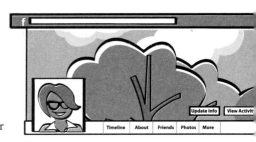

Members typically include a photo and some basic information, such as where they work, where they live, their educational background, their hobbies, their interests, and any websites they run.

What about privacy on Facebook?

You have choices here. Your profile can remain private until you approve someone as your Facebook friend. Or, your profile can be public, meaning anyone can find you and view everything on your site. (I would not recommend this.)

✗ Faux Pas

In the summer of 2010, a Michigan nurse was fired for venting on Facebook. Like many others, she was upset when a local policeman was shot to death pursuing a suspect. As part of her duties as a nurse, she treated the shooter. The problem resulted when she posted on Facebook that she came "face to face" with a "cop killer" and hoped he "rotted in hell." She was fired because she disseminated protected health information about a patient. She made it easy to identify the patient without revealing his name.

How can Facebook benefit nurses?

You can find many groups that pertain to nursing on Facebook. This is a great way to connect and share information with other nurses. On Facebook, you can "follow" a group. For example, you can "follow" the American Nurses Association on Facebook to get the latest news and connect with other nurses. The following box offers suggestions of groups you can follow on Facebook. These groups

These groups can help keep nurses up to date. They can also affect your (and your employer's) ability to provide care by enabling you to learn a new procedure or strategy and share it with your nursing colleagues.

In addition to following a group, you can create a group of your own by building a special page for it. You can determine if anyone is allowed to follow (open membership) your page or if someone needs to be invited to follow (closed membership).

Facebook Resources for Nurses

- American Nurses Association
- Johns Hopkins Medicine
- May Clinic
- Nurse.com
- Nurse rounds

Do you have any etiquette tips for using Facebook?

Yes. Here are some of the basics:

- Don't discuss patients with your friends and followers, even if the patient is someone you know.

- To engage with your friends and followers, post entertaining content regularly.

- Make your friends and followers feel welcome on your page.

- If you want to post often in one day, spread out your posts over several hours.

- Respond to all comments—good and bad.

If I am using Facebook to connect with friends and family, should I be concerned about business implications?

Yes. What you post can get you fired. For example, people have called in sick to work and then posted photos of themselves at a casino. How silly is that?

Twitter

Why is Twitter so popular?

Twitter (www.twitter.com) is all about quick and easy conversation. Its simplicity is the reason for its popularity and amazing success. Twitter is a microblogging application that asks the question, "What's happening?" Posts or responses must be 140 characters or less. Users can post updates, or tweets, as often as they want via a mobile phone, instant messaging, or a web browser. Posts are displayed on the user's technology of choice (text message, website, Twitter account, Facebook page, etc.).

What is the point of responding to the question, "What's happening?"

If your response is, "I'm eating pizza," there is no point. However, when used strategically, Twitter can help you to connect with others,

✗ Faux Pas

Sadie, age 23, started a fire in Oregon because her firefighter friends were out of work. Two days after the fire began, she went on Facebook and posted an entry stating, "Like my fire?" This post led to her identity and arrest. This shows that you never know who will read your posts.

✗ Faux Pas

A former healthcare worker was receiving disability payments because she claimed to be incapacitated by back problems from a work-related injury. Her disability payments stopped, however, when pictures of her on Facebook showed her dancing while on cruise in the Mediterranean. You never know who will share your information!

make announcements, build brands, provide project updates, and promote services and products. Many professional conferences encourage participants to tweet about what they are learning and who is speaking. This is valuable PR.

What are some examples of how organizations use Twitter?

Here are some examples to illustrate how Twitter is widely used and very helpful:

- Healthcare agencies tweet flu statistics.

- Nursing conferences encourage attendees to tweet and tell what they are learning.

- Whole Foods Market uses Twitter to provide product information.

- NASA uses Twitter to provide updates on space shuttle missions.

- News agencies, such as the BBC, use Twitter to disseminate breaking news.

- Reporters and television newscasters often ask for and read comments sent in on Twitter.

- Political campaigns use Twitter for publicity.

- The Los Angeles Fire Department uses Twitter to get up-to-the second information on where fires are breaking out and where people are trapped.

How do I join Twitter?

Signing up for Twitter is free and easy. Just visit www.twitter.com and follow the prompts to sign up. After you sign up, you can subscribe to different Twitter feeds to receive updates. You can follow the Twitter feeds of anyone you choose—for example, doctors, nurses, movie stars, athletes, authors, newscasters, heads of state, medical centers, friends, and family members.

The following box contains good Twitter feeds for nurses.

Twitter Feeds of Interest to Nurses

- **@Womenshealth:** The Office of Women's Health, part of the U.S. Department of Health and Human Services
- **@NavigateNursing:** A resource for nurses seeking to create healthier work environments
- **@RNCentral:** Nursing education, news, and healthy living tips
- **@TheLancet:** The world's leading general medical journal
- **@NursingWorld:** ANA Government Affairs, leading the fight for nurses on Capitol Hill

What is the basic vocabulary associated with Twitter?

Here are some of the basics terms (Safko & Brake, 2009):

- **Tweet:** Something that someone posts on Twitter.
- **Twitterer:** Someone who uses Twitter to send tweets, or posts.
- **The Twitosphere:** A name for the Twitter community.
- **Mistweet:** A tweet posted by accident or that you wish you could take back.

How is Twitter different from sending an email or blogging?

Because of the limit on the size of a tweet, Twitter is used to update networks with information that is more casual than an email and more concise than a blog (Scott, 2009).

What are some etiquette guidelines for nurses who use Twitter?

Here are some guidelines to follow:

- Respect patient privacy issues.

- Treat your Twitter posts as though they will be read by your parents and managers.

- Avoid sharing too much personal information.

- Don't tweet about the minutiae of your day.

- Don't tweet profanity or anything unprofessional.

- Use the At Reply (@reply) function to reply on Twitter. To do this, hover over the tweet and click the At Reply option. After you complete your @reply, click the Tweet button to post it.

- Retweet posts you find interesting.

- Don't just watch. Be part of the conversation.

- If sharing an article, include a link to the original source.

- Upload a photo of yourself to differentiate yourself from spammers.

- Be gracious to those who promote your tweets.

- Offer content that is a mix of information, thoughts, recommendations, and resources.

- Respond to questions and comments quickly.

- Ask questions, provide answers, share news, and provide links.

- Don't feel you have to follow everyone who follows you.

- Use pithy sayings.

- Keep your comments positive.
- Don't tweet anything negative about your workplace.

What if I get tired of following someone on Twitter?

Simply unfollow that person. When content shared by that person is no longer relevant, it's time to opt out.

> Social media has the word "me" in it, so people tweet about themselves.
>
> —George Takei

What if Twitter has overwhelmed my life balance?

Back off and unfollow. Moderation is the key.

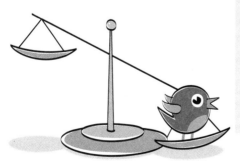

X Faux Pas

An employee of an advertising company had a huge contract with a car company in Detroit. When he tweeted negative comments about Detroit drivers, he thought he was using his personal account. However, he was on the company's account. He got fired, and his company lost the contract with the car company (Pachter, 2013).

X Faux Pas

During the 2012 London Olympics, a Greek athlete was kicked off the team for tweets mocking African immigrants. Also, a Swiss athlete was banned from the Olympics for a racist tweet about South Koreans. Rude and unkind behaviors have consequences and affect careers.

✓ Good Idea!

A nurse manager went online to find a hotel room in New York City for a nursing conference. She was disappointed that no rooms were available in Midtown. She sent a tweet to her network for help. Within minutes, she heard from a number of people with suggestions and got a reservation at a boutique hotel in downtown Manhattan.

Is Twitter valuable for networking?

Yes. Twitter is a great way to build your network. Twitter also has a job search component to help people find jobs. Here are some ideas to help expand your network:

- Follow interesting people. Use a Twitter search to find people by name, profession, or interest.

- Share information, such as job postings and links to journal articles.

- Populate your profile on Twitter, including links to your website, blog, or other forms of social media.

- Have Twitter search your Google, Yahoo!, and AOL accounts to help you find people you already know on the site.

- Use Twellow (www.twellow.com) to find Twitter users in a certain geographical area.

- Follow conversations for a time and then join in.

- If you are interested in connecting with someone, retweet some of his or her posts before introducing yourself.

- Send tweets via your mobile phone with the Twitter mobile app, available free for iPhone, Galaxy, and Windows Phone.

- Don't spam.

Google Plus

What is Google+?

Google+ (plus.google.com) is another way of keeping in touch with selected groups of people using circles of connection. As an example, you could have circles for your work friends, your college friends, and your neighbors. Circles are used to compartmentalize your followers so you can share targeted information to the right group.

You can post text, photos, links, video, polls, and events. You can also join communities and share ideas. You or your business can be easily found by someone doing a search, using Google+, or using any mobile device.

If you go online, you will find numerous tutorials explaining how to use this service.

What are some etiquette tips for using Google+?

Here are some basic tips:

- Don't post anything unprofessional.

- Don't violate patient privacy.

- When sharing a post, add you own commentary first.

- Share valuable information and include people in the conversation by mentioning them.

- Format your posts. Make them easier to read with bold, italics, etc.

- Use *hat tips* when sharing the work of others. People want to be recognized for their work.

Can I block someone from contacting me on Google+?

Yes. When you block someone, that person will not be able to see anything you post. You will be removed from that person's circles, and he or she will be removed from yours. In addition, the person will not be informed that he or she has been blocked. (Of course, if the person knows your email address, he or she can still contact you by email.)

LinkedIn

Why do professionals join LinkedIn?

It is important to separate your private life from your work life. LinkedIn (www.linkedin.com) enables users to do just that. This site is an online professional contact database for business professionals that allows members to create a profile and link with contacts they know and trust.

LinkedIn helps users keep in touch with people with whom they have worked in the past, even if they have changed jobs or switched positions. This site is great for networking and can connect the right person to the right contact at the right time. Nurses use LinkedIn to connect with other nursing professionals, highlight their achievements and to find job opportunities. These are LinkedIn's best benefits for nurses.

How do I get started with LinkedIn?

Go to www.linkedin.com and set up a free account. You will be asked some questions (for example, about your education and degrees) and will be prompted to provide information about your work history. Include your current contact information and keep people up-to-date on your accomplishments. Don't hesitate to mention honors and awards. Add your professional "elevator speech" about who you are and what you do as a summary paragraph. (See

Chapter 1, "Making Your Acquaintance," for help crafting an elevator speech.) Also include your photo. If you don't add a photo, your
profile will feature a nonspecific silhouette, which is not very entic-
ing.

How do I connect with others on LinkedIn?

You can use LinkedIn's basic email invitation message to connect
with others. For best results, personalize the message by reminding
people of how you are connected. For example, you might write, "It
was nice being on the panel with you at the AORN conference in
Boston."

LinkedIn Group Suggestions for Nurses

- American Nurses Association
- ADVANCE for Nurses
- Nursing Jobs
- RN Network
- Nurse Practitioner
- Nursing Beyond the Bedside
- Oncology Nursing Society
- Flight Nurses

Should I ask people to recommend me?

Yes. If people haven't recommended you independently, you can ask
for recommendations from those who know you and value what
you do. You should also provide recommendations for others who
have done good work. Recommendations are a two-way street.

A quick way to acknowledge others is to use LinkedIn's endorsement feature. It is another way to highlight someone's expertise and
skills—for example, public speaking, leadership, nursing, staff development, and so on.

When should I post on LinkedIn?

Keep your profile up-to-date. Post when you publish an article or book, or when you receive a new position or award. Also, join groups that are beneficial to your career and contribute to the groups' discussions by sharing your knowledge and experience.

What are some etiquette tips for using LinkedIn?

On LinkedIn, it's critical that you present yourself as an articulate professional. Consider the following points:

- Keep your updates related to professional matters.

- Don't forget patient privacy issues.

- Save daily life updates for Facebook and Twitter.

- Once connected, send a welcome message to build connections.

- Don't send a mass request for recommendations.

- Send requests for recommendations only to people who know you and can vouch for your work.

- Use groups as a place to contribute valuable information.

- Don't use groups to promote your business.

- Compare your resume and your online profile. Make sure there is not a disconnect between the two.

Do employers use LinkedIn?

They sure do. In fact, it is one of the first things they check for background information on job applicants. Employers can use LinkedIn to find out where candidates worked and for whom. They may have contacts who worked at the same place and be able to get inside information about your job expertise and professionalism.

What are the different levels of connection on LinkedIn?

There are different levels of connection on LinkedIn. These levels are based on how well two people know each other. The levels are as follows:

- **Primary or first-degree connections:** These are people you know directly and to whom you are immediately linked. These connections can be viewed and contacted anytime.

- **Second-degree connections:** These are contacts known by people you know.

- **Third-degree connections:** These are contacts of your second-degree connections.

Additional degree connections follow the same pattern.

Your list of connections increases exponentially based on the connections of your contacts. Through your connections, you increase the likelihood that someone you know can facilitate a desired introduction for you.

Connecting via a personal connection is easier than making a cold call. For example, suppose you are writing a book and want to get an endorsement from a well-known nursing leader. One of your connections is connected to someone who is connected to the nursing leader. It may well be that your connection can arrange an introduction for you. That is the beauty of LinkedIn!

TIP

First impressions begin long before the interview process.

Instagram

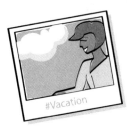

What is Instagram?

Instagram (www.instagram.com) facilitates photo sharing. It is a fun way to share your life with friends though pictures. It has filters that can transform your photos into snapshots that look professional. You can snap a photo, transform the feel and look of the photo, add comments, and then share.

What about privacy?

By default, all photos on Instagram are public. This makes them visible to anyone using Instagram or on the Instagram website. Additionally, if your account is public, anyone can subscribe to follow your photos. However, you can control who sees your photos if you choose the private option.

Instagram was acquired by Facebook in 2012. However, you still can decide whether to post your Instagram photos on Facebook.

How do I find friends on Instagram?

Instagram has a Find Friends feature that can help you locate others with Instagram accounts by using your contact list, through third-party social media sites, or by searching names and usernames on Instagram.

What are some etiquette tips for using Instagram?

Here are some basic guidelines:

- Don't *overgram*—that is, post too many pictures.
- Don't take pictures of patients.

- Don't post pictures that make fun of difficult patients.

- Keep your posts clean.

- Avoid selfies, food, and family photos.

- Don't repost someone's photo without permission.

- Don't ask people to follow you.

Instagram Accounts for Nurses and Nursing Students

- **@NursesOfInstagram:** This account includes inspirational quotes, humor, and style tips for scrubs.

- **@FindNursingSchools:** Here, you'll see tips for finding the right school for you.

- **@NursingLOL:** This account will make you laugh out loud with its jokes and cartoons.

- **@ExploreNursing:** This account shares information about the nursing profession and nursing shortage, mixed with inspirational and humorous quotes.

- **@TheDrOzShow:** This account promotes highlights from the Dr. Oz Show.

Pinterest

What is Pinterest and how is it used?

Pinterest (www.pinterest.com) is a digital scrapbook of photos and images on a variety of topics. Examples include gifts, holidays, fashion, humor, quotes, recipes, clothing, parties, camping, home decorating, fitness, weddings, and crafts. You can find ideas for your projects and interests on Pinterest.

What are some etiquette tips for using Pinterest?

Here are some guidelines (DelBalzo, 2014):

- Pin directly from the source material. That way, you give credit to the originator of the content.

- Use high-quality images.

- Spread your pins out over the day. Don't repin for one straight hour.

- Don't use images unrelated to your content. That is only confusing.

- Make sure the images on your website are easily pinnable.

- Make sure your links are in order. Check this on a regular basis.

Blogging

The tipping point for "wait and see" [about blogs] is swinging like a metronome, toward "better do something now."

–Debbie Weil

Where did the term *blog* come from?

The word *blog* comes from *weblog*, which is an online journal. A blog is a website maintained by someone with regular entries or posts that include ideas, thoughts, and commentaries. Photos, graphics, audio, and video can be part of the posts (Safko & Brake, 2009).

Blogs can provide content about a specific subject or can act as a personal journal. For example, you might create a blog that focuses on sharing tips for patients with diabetes mellitus, sharing gluten-free recipes, your volunteer service in Haiti, or your cross-country biking trip.

Can blogs benefit patients?

They sure can. For example, as mentioned, a blog with tips for patients with diabetes would be a good resource for some patients. Or, patients with fibromyalgia could benefit from reading blogs by others who suffer from the same condition. As a nurse, you could help patients find blogs of interest. For example, at the blog PatientsLikeMe (http://blog.patientslikeme.com), people with different conditions share their health experiences, find patients like them, and learn how to take control of their healthcare.

> **TIP**
>
> **Focus your blog on a particular theme and a target audience.**

What are some of the key features of blogs?

Here are some features that have contributed to the popularity of blogs:

- Blogs permit two-way communication. Readers can interact with the author.

- Starting a blog is simple.

- Blogs can help position the author as a thought leader.

- Adding a post to a blog is as easy as sending an email.

How are blogs different from websites?

Blogs are more engaging than static websites. Here are some of the main differences:

- Blogs are interactive.

- Blogs are typically written in a conversational tone.

- Blogs are easily created. No technical expertise is needed.

- Blogs are updated frequently.

- Blogs get higher rankings in search engines than static websites.

- Blogs can alert readers whenever something new is added, without an email.

What kind of software is needed to start a blog?

There are a lot of free choices. WordPress.com (www.wordpress.com) and Blogger (www.blogger.com) are very popular. Setting up a blog is easy and can be done in a few minutes. Other forms of software are available for purchase with monthly fees.

Blogs are often misperceived by people who don't read them.

–David M. Scott

How often should blogs be updated?

This is up to you. Maintaining a blog requires dedication and effort. You can post daily, weekly, or less often. The time you invest is related to the purpose of your blog and your priorities.

That being said, don't let your blog go quiet without an explanation. If you need to take a break, tell your readers you are taking a hiatus and when to expect you back.

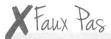 **Faux Pas**

In a *60 Minutes* broadcast in September of 2004, documents were presented that were critical of President George W. Bush's service in the National Guard. The documents were presented as authentic, but had not been properly vetted. When bloggers questioned the authenticity of the documents, veteran newscaster Dan Rather dismissed them as a bunch of "geeks in pajamas." Ignoring the bloggers cost him his job. Had he taken them seriously and investigated the documents, he would have concluded that they were false (Scott, 2009).

What is the best length for a blog post?

For the most part, posts are short. Lengths vary. A good goal is under 1,000 words.

How do blog readers know when I post a new entry?

One of the essential features of a blog is a Really Simple Syndication (RSS) feed, or web feed. Readers receive an automatic update every time content is added. Because email is not needed, the updates are not lost in a clogged inbox or blocked by spam. Blog entries are displayed in reverse chronological order. The most recent post appears at the top of the page.

What are some tips for boosting my nursing career by blogging?

Here are some suggestions to help you boost your career by blogging (Pagana, K. D., 2013d; Safko & Brake, 2009):

- Write as if you are talking to your nursing colleagues or patients.

- Be yourself and let your personality shine through.

- Focus your blog around a certain mission or theme, such as healthy eating.

- Share your expertise on a topic, such as joint replacement.

- Offer unique and valuable information.

- Reflect on current practices or healthcare issues.

- Follow HIPAA guidelines for patient confidentiality.

- Post often.

- Use catchy post titles.

- Ask open-ended questions.

- Use images in your posts.

- Link to other blog posts.

- Link to your other social profiles.

- Read other blogs.

- When your post receives a comment, reply to further the conversation.

How much information should a blog include about its author?

Background information helps to establish your credibility. It is good idea to have an "About" page with a photo, biography, affiliations, and other relevant information.

How do I find a blog for an area of interest or particular topic?

Some good places to start include Google (www.google.com), Blog Search Engine (www.blogsearchengine.org),

Yahoo! (www.yahoo.com), and Technorati (www.technorati.com), which is the most comprehensive source of information.

Blogs for Nurses

- **ER Nurses Care:** http://ernursescare.blogspot.com/
- **DiversityNursing Blog:** http://blog.diversitynursing.com/blog
- **Innovative Nurse:** http://innovativenurse.com/
- **The Nursing Site Blog:** http://www.thenursingsiteblog.com/
- **The Nerdy Nurse:** http://thenerdynurse.com/
- **Off the Charts:** http://ajnoffthecharts.com/

Eventually, most business will use blogs to communicate with customers, suppliers, and employers because it's two-way and more satisfying.

–Bill Gates

How do I determine if a blog is credible?

Remember, anyone can create a blog. Don't believe everything you read in a blog. Blogs build credibility the same way as any other source of information. They need to earn your trust.

TIP

Self-promotion gets old to blog readers. Minimize it.

Is it OK to pitch products or services on my blog?

That is a turnoff to readers. The goal of your blog should be to create a demand for your services though demonstrated expertise, relevance, and information versus solicitation. Pull the audience in; don't push them out. If you have books to sell, it is better to have a link to your website or shopping cart.

How do organizations and businesses use blogs?

Here are some examples of ways organizations and businesses use blogs:

- For organizational leaders to communicate with customers or patients

- For employees to communicate with customers

- For customers or patients to provide unsolicited feedback

- For employers to share information with employees via an intranet

- To attract the best employees

- To attract new customers or patients

- To advocate specific issues (such as health insurance)

How can a blog be used within an organization?

A blog can be placed on an intranet and made available to employees. Blogs can transform a static, one-way, top-down intranet into a dynamic, interactive tool for collaboration. Here are some examples of internal uses of blogs within an organization:

- News blogs (achievements, announcements, birthdays, etc.)
- CEO blogs (to explain financial decisions and ask for ideas)
- Project coordination
- Client feedback and satisfaction surveys
- Interdepartmental team blogs (to connect those who don't work in the same area)

How do I deal with comments on a blog?

Blogging software offers several options with respect to commenting. One option is not to allow comments, but that eliminates a popular feature of blogs. Another option is to permit comments that are not subject to your approval. Or, you can opt to approve comments before they appear on the blog.

Many bloggers use the approval process to prevent users from posting inappropriate comments on their blog. However, you should post comments that show disagreement because healthy debate is an indicator of a well-read blog (Scott, 2009). If only rosy comments are posted, credibility will suffer.

What are *blooks*?

Many bloggers have published books based on their original blogs. These are called *blooks*. For example, a compilation of blogs about nursing leadership could end up as a blook. A hospice nurse who blogs about his or her experiences may have the foundation for a book on death and dying.

Frequently Asked Questions

 How do nurse recruiters use social networking sites when hiring staff?

Many employers use these sites to do background and character checks. They also scan them for questionable posts, videos, or photographs.

 Is it OK to comment on Facebook about my patients as long as I don't mention them by name?

No. Check your healthcare organization's policy about social media. Any information about a patient that allows another to recognize the patient is a breach of confidentiality. This could result in job termination, fines, penalties, and jail time.

 If my manager or chief nursing officer (CNO) sends me a Facebook friend request, should I accept it?

You are under no obligation to accept. Many people restrict Facebook to their friends and family. Consider sending the person an invitation to LinkedIn. Another option is to accept the invitation and use your privacy settings to limit what sections of your profile your manager or CNO can see.

 Should I give someone an explanation if I defriend him or her on Facebook?

That is not necessary. Facebook doesn't send out notifications when someone is defriended. So, the person may never know. He or she will just stop receiving your updates in his or her news feed. If the person is someone you run into often, you may tell him or her you are cutting back your use of Facebook or limiting it to family only.

When traveling, is it a good idea detail my travel plans on social media?

No. Many people's homes have been burglarized because "friends" knew they were away. Some burglars have selected houses based on Facebook updates.

How confident can I be about using privacy settings on my social media sites?

Don't take any chances! Remember that privacy settings do not guarantee that something you post will remain private. Your link may be shared by a friend, and then by a friend, and so on. That's how posts go viral.

When signing up for a social media site, do I have to give all the information requested?

No. Only provide information you feel comfortable sharing with others.

Can blogs increase traffic to a website?

Yes. Search engines love blogs. They generate higher rankings on Google than websites.

Who should I talk to if I want to post information about a job or the latest news from our hospital on social media?

Check the hospital's social media policy. You can also discuss this with someone in marketing or human resources. If you want to post information about a job, make sure the positon is open to the public and not just for internal candidates.

TAKE-AWAY TIPS

✓ Social media is redefining the way people communicate and do business.

✓ Don't post anything on social media that you would be embarrassed to see on the front page of a newspaper.

✓ It takes a long time to develop trust and build a following on Twitter. It takes only one tweet to alienate all of your followers.

✓ Never share your passwords. If you do, change the password.

✓ Blogs provide both experts and wannabes with an easy way to make their voices heard. Don't trust everything you read.

✓ The value of social media is underestimated by those who haven't bothered to learn about it.

✓ Plan time to explore and learn about unfamiliar forms of social media.

✓ Have a consistent image across all of your online platforms.

✓ Social media is here to stay. You may appear out of touch if you don't stay up-to-date with it.

✓ Play nice, say thank you, and foster relationships with social media.

8

Mingling Among the Cocktail Set

Juggling Drinks and Hors d'Oeuvres at Corporate Events

Do you:

Feel anxious and wonder if you should attend the holiday party?

Know what to wear?

Know how to initiate and sustain small talk?

Know how much alcohol you can drink and still act appropriately?

Know how to handle drinks and hors d'oeuvres?

Wonder if you should bring a gift?

Have a spouse who does not want to attend your business function?

Wonder if you should send a thank-you note afterward?

These are important concerns for new and even seasoned employees. Inappropriate behavior at cocktail parties, receptions, retirement parties, award ceremonies, and other corporate events can undo years of good impressions. Your career aspirations can be enhanced or limited by your behavior as you navigate these potentially disastrous social gatherings.

Etiquette is what you are doing and saying when people are looking and listening. What you are thinking is your business.

–Virginia Cary Hudson

Greetings and Courtesy

Is it really necessary to attend my unit or department party?

Yes, unless you want to be remembered as the person who snubbed your colleagues by not attending. Your absence at an annual function will be noted.

Attending the party shows you are a team player and gives you a chance to get to know co-workers in a less formal setting. Think of the office party as part of your job. If this is not your idea of a good time, consider it work. Put on your best attitude and go. If you are unable to attend due to a scheduling conflict, let your host and others know why.

What should I do if I have accepted an invitation and discover at the last minute that I cannot attend?

Make every effort to contact the host to let him or her know why you will miss the event. Here are some other suggestions (Rickenbacher, 2004):

- Call the location of the event and leave a message with the banquet manager or maître d' to be passed to the host.
- Send a handwritten note the next day explaining your absence.
- Call the host the next day. Apologize and explain your situation.

Is a business party a time to relax and let loose?

No. It is a test of your social skills and your level of sophistication. Your interpersonal skills, including your treatment of the waitstaff, are on display.

One of the biggest blunders at a business function is alcohol abuse. You can undo months and years of good impressions by excessive drinking. The key point to remember is that business behavior is the number-one concern at the gathering (Pagana, K. D., 2006c).

Why are many people uncomfortable attending social events?

In recent years, teenagers and children have faced unprecedented demands on their time from school and extracurricular activities. In addition, most families are two-earner families, with both parents working full-time jobs. As a result, fewer people have time to focus on learning social graces—including small talk. This contributes to the anxiety that many people feel in formal or business functions.

For many people, including nurses on the job, time is so precious that we practice getting to the point and the task at hand as quickly as possible so we can move on to the next point or task. However, many businesses expect employees to have the social skills needed to make them a competent representative for the organization.

No matter your age, social skills are important for career advancement. Learn them! In addition to this book, numerous resources are available. In addition, many community, business, and school organizations offer courses that teach these skills.

When should I arrive for a company party?

It is best to arrive on time. Do not be more than 15 to 20 minutes late (Post, 2014). A late entrance will make people think you are rude. Punctuality is expected more at a business event than a social event.

On the other hand, don't arrive early. This can be awkward for the host if he or she is not quite ready for the party.

Should I bring family or a partner to a business event?

If they are invited and you would like them to attend, that is fine. Just be aware that their actions and dress will reflect on you. You should brief them ahead of time on proper dress, conversational topics, key people, and expected behavior.

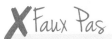 **✗ Faux Pas**

Bill was being honored at a cocktail party for receiving a national award. His family members were invited. His sisters stuck together and made no effort to interact with anyone else. Unfortunately, they lost the opportunity to meet Bill's colleagues. They could have asked, "How do you know Bill?" as a conversation starter and met a lot of nice people. Instead, they came across as backward and socially awkward. They were not an asset to Bill in his goal for career advancement.

Do you have any recommendations for presenting oneself professionally at a corporate event?

Think of a corporate event as a great opportunity to expand your network and make new friends. At this type of event, you can practice your skills related to introductions, handshaking, remembering names, conversations, and networking. Here are some guidelines (Brody, 2005; Pachter, 2013; Sabath, 2010):

- Smile and be friendly to everyone.

- Avoid clustering in small groups with people in your department.

- Introduce yourself to people you don't know.

- Take the time and effort to get acquainted with new people.

- Spend more time listening than talking.

- Ask open-ended questions.

- Keep the conversational topics accessible to everyone.

- Minimize "shop talk" during social gatherings.

- Be sure to greet senior management. Use engaging small talk.

- If you don't call people by their first names at work, don't start at the social event.

- Don't take or make any phone calls.

- Treat the servers with respect.

- Don't act bored. Be aware of your body language.

- Stay for an appropriate amount of time.

- Thank your hosts before leaving.

✓ Good Idea!

As the new VP of nursing, Felix was looking forward to getting to know the administrative team better at the annual holiday gala. As part of his preparation for the event, he found out as much as he could about the people who were going to be there. Because of this preparation, he had no trouble fitting in with the team. He used small talk to initiate conversations and begin to develop working relationships.

What is the dress code for a corporate event?

The key word here is *corporate*. Make sure you dress appropriately for the function by checking the invitation or calling the host for guidelines. Remember, the way you dress when out with friends and family may not be suitable for a work function. Dress up. It is always best to err on the more formal side. Your effort will be apparent and reflect favorably on you.

TIP

Women should avoid clothes that are too tight, too short, and too sexy.

How do I deal with gossip?

Avoid gossipers. It is not enough to abstain from gossip. Silence can be a form of participation. Excuse yourself and remove yourself from the situation.

If there are no place cards on the dinner tables, can I sit wherever I want?

Yes. But be sure you are not sitting at the host's table. If people are already seated at a table, ask them for permission to join them. For example, you might say, "Do you mind if I join you?" or "Are these chairs available?" A chair tilted against the table means that place is taken.

If I am invited to a party at someone's house, should I bring a gift?

Yes. The host expends a lot of time and money to put on a party. A small gift expresses your appreciation and gratitude. The gift does not have to be expensive, but it should be nicely wrapped. Some suggestions include a bottle of wine, fragrant candles, or a box of chocolates. A small gift basket with jams or gourmet foods is also a nice option. Attach a card so the host will know who brought it. If you bring wine, do not expect the host to serve it at the party. If you bring flowers, put them in a vase before giving them to the host.

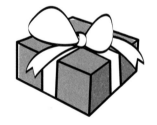

Should I send a thank-you note after the occasion?

Yes. If you want to show appreciation, demonstrate good manners, and be remembered, send a thank-you note. This should be a handwritten note.

Small Talk

Why is small talk important at a corporate function?

Small talk is essential for starting conversations until you find a common area of interest. It is a valuable tool for breaking the ice and making people feel comfortable. Small talk is a gateway to new relationships and vital for maintaining established relationships.

If you have trouble getting started with small talk, try using the OAR approach to help your conversation:

- **Observe:** Make an observation—for example, "It looks like this new restaurant drew a large crowd."

- **Ask questions:** For example, you might ask, "How is your daughter doing on the swim team?"

- **Reveal:** Reveal something about yourself. For example, you might say, "Now that I've been at Susquehanna Health for 3 years, it is nice to know most of the people here."

How do I know what topics are safe for conversation?

Avoid controversial topics, especially religion and politics. Don't discuss salary, medical problems, or personal misfortunes. You can safely discuss weather, sports, traffic, travel, movies, and books. Avoid off-color jokes.

During a social event, don't discuss work problems. Avoid medical jargon. If a conversation turns to work, change the subject by saying something like, "I heard you mention a trip earlier. Where are you are planning to go?"

Don't forget to protect patient privacy in your conversations. It is unethical and illegal to discuss patients outside of the healthcare team.

✗ Faux Pas

Joe invited his friend Patrick to play golf with him and two of his colleagues in a fundraiser for a new cancer treatment center. Although Patrick was a good golfer, Joe regretted inviting him to the tournament because Patrick talked the entire time about his medical problems. He dominated the conversation and put a damper on the golf outing.

How do I exit gracefully from conversations?

This is a key component of networking at corporate events. Your goal is to meet several people, not to spend the entire time speaking with one person. Simply excuse yourself and say something like, "It has been great talking with you. I'll let you have time to speak to others." Or, "It was a pleasure meeting you. Will you excuse me while I touch base with some other colleagues?"

Alcoholic Beverages and Hors d'Oeuvres

Always do sober what you said you'd do drunk. That will teach you to keep your mouth shut.

–Ernest Hemingway

Do you have any suggestions for drinking at a corporate event?

Limit yourself to one or two drinks. This can be a challenge when the drinks are free and the liquor is high quality. Don't think you need to drink to be part of the group. Stop drinking when you reach your limit, and switch to a nonalcoholic beverage. You do not want to be remembered for any colorful or inappropriate behavior. You will be held accountable for your actions.

What is the best way to hold drinks and hors d'oeuvres?

The best way to hold drinks and hors d'oeuvres is to handle them separately. It is very awkward to hold a drink in one hand and food in the other. This restricts your ability to shake hands. Remember, the purpose of the event is to socialize, not to eat and drink. Don't be hungry and thirsty when you arrive at the event.

TIP

Remember, business behavior is the number one item on the agenda at any business event.

✗ Faux Pas

Justin was at a corporate out-of-town dinner with his team. His boss offered wine. Justin, along with the rest of the team, accepted the offer of a glass. When the wine was brought to the table, a co-worker who had been drinking before and during the meal grabbed the glass the waiter had offered to the boss to taste and approve. In addition, she was the only one to order an after-dinner drink. Everyone at the table was embarrassed for her. Her career with the hospital was short-lived, as this type of inappropriate behavior was also demonstrated—in less dramatic ways—in her everyday work.

What do I do with the toothpick used to serve food from a serving tray?

Don't put the toothpick back on the tray. Put the toothpick in your napkin or on a tray used to collect empty glasses and plates.

Avoiding Buffet Blunders

- Put your food selections on a plate.
- Don't snack over the buffet table.
- Move away from the table to eat your food.
- Don't complain about the food. Just select food you like and pass on food you do not want.
- Don't double-dip your food in sauces.

Wine Service

What is the proper way for the host to handle wine at a meal?

Assuming the event is taking place in a restaurant, here's the proper way for the host to handle wine:

1. The host orders a bottle of wine.

2. The server presents the wine bottle to the host.

3. The host examines the label to make certain it is the correct type and vintage.

4. The server removes the seal, extracts the cork, and places the cork on the table.

5. The host looks at the cork to make sure it is in good condition.

6. The server pours a small amount of wine into a glass for the host to sample.

7. The host swirls the wine in a small motion, sniffs the wine, and takes a small sip.

8. If the wine tastes good, the guests are served prior to the host.

9. If the wine tastes off or has a musky odor, the problem is reported to the server. The server or wine steward may taste to confirm. A replacement bottle will be provided.

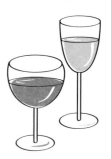

TIP

It is hard to be polite when you are starved. Eat something before the event.

Is there a different type of wine glass used for white and red wine?

Yes. A red wine glass has a short stem and a large bowl. Red wine is served at room temperature. Hold the glass close to the bowl.

A white wine glass has a longer stem and a smaller bowl. White wine is served chilled. Hold the glass by the stem to avoid warming the wine with the heat from your hand.

✔ Good Idea!

Theresa was attending her first corporate cocktail party. She didn't want to make a bad impression by heading straight to the buffet to get something to eat, so she ate something before she arrived. Once there, she ordered a soda with a lime, which she carried in her left hand, leaving her right hand free to shake hands. She met many new people and had a great time at the party. She was very savvy and conducted herself with charm, which her managers noticed. When she got home, she and her husband shared a bottle of wine and discussed the party.

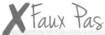 Faux Pas

Dave made sure he was appropriately dressed for the office party at a nice country club. He limited his drinking to one glass of wine. However, he stood by the shrimp bar and ate more than 20 pieces of shrimp. He forgot that the main purpose of the event was to mingle and network. His co-workers did not forget this incident. They endlessly teased him and made him the butt of many shrimp jokes.

How much money should I spend on a bottle of wine?

A sensible guideline is to spend as much on a bottle of wine as the cost of one complete dinner. Be careful, however. Wine prices vary from a few dollars to hundreds of dollars.

How can I ask the wine steward to suggest a wine in my price range?

Point to some prices on the menu and ask for suggestions.

In which hand should I hold my glass of wine?

Keep your drink in your left hand so your right hand is free for shaking hands. You don't want your right hand to be cold and damp.

Should I tip the bartender?

If it is a cash bar where you pay for your drinks, you should tip the bartender. At most formal affairs, gratuities are built into the waitstaff's fees (Post, 2014).

How do I select wine?

Red wine is usually recommended with red meat, although this rule is not carved in stone. White wine is usually recommended with white meat or fish. However, these are just suggestions. You can ask the wine steward to make suggestions to complement your meal choices.

Popular examples of red wines include merlot, zinfandel, shiraz, and pinot noir. Popular whites include chardonnay and sauvignon blanc (Pachter, 2013).

How do I know how many bottles of wine to order for a group of people?

As a rule of thumb, order one bottle for three people (Pachter, 2013).

Beer Drinking

If I am drinking beer at a corporate event, should I use a glass?

Yes. Pour it into a pilsner glass. Stay away from plastic glasses unless no others are available.

Do you have any suggestions for drinking beer at a cocktail party or dinner?

Yes. Pour the beer into a large glass that will hold the entire can or bottle. This avoids the need to put beer cans or bottles on the table.

At a formal party, it looks classier to carry a glass of beer instead of a bottle or can. However, if you are at function where the hosts are drinking out of a bottle or can, feel free to do the same.

TIP

If you have a question about how to handle a drink or food, follow the lead of your host or those in the position you aspire to.

If I am at a ballgame with my boss and colleagues, is it OK to drink a beer?

Yes, if you can handle yourself in an appropriate manner. Remember, your behavior at the ballgame will be remembered in the boardroom.

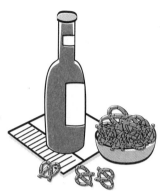

Tasteful Toasting

Why do people make toasts?

The custom of toasting to health dates back to ancient Greece, when a sip of wine was taken to demonstrate that the wine was not poisoned. Splashing wine from cup to cup was also a safeguard against poisoning. Today, a toast is used to recognize a special occasion (Whitmore, 2005).

How can I make a memorable toast?

Keep it simple and short. It is a toast, not a roast. Prepare ahead of time so you do not fumble for the appropriate words.

Can anyone propose the first toast at an event?

The host or hostess should propose the first toast. If there is a guest of honor, the host or hostess should toast the person. The honored guest should respond with a toast. Other guests are then free to make toasts.

If the guest of honor is being toasted, does he or she take a drink?

No. The person being honored should smile and say thank you. It is considered bad form to drink to oneself.

If I do not drink alcohol, can I participate in a toast?

Yes. You can toast with a nonalcoholic beverage or water. You can also raise a glass of wine to your lips without tasting it.

Avoiding Toasting Blunders

- Don't read a toast. However, you may glance at your written notes.
- Don't clink glasses.
- Don't tap the rim of a glass to get everyone's attention.
- Don't toast yourself.
- Don't feel you need to drink alcohol to propose a toast.
- Don't raise your glass above eye level.

Frequently Asked Questions

How soon should I respond to an RSVP?

It is best to respond within a few days to a week. Definitely respond before the date indicated. The RSVP means you have to respond one way or another. Don't make the host have to call you for your response. If you decline, include a brief reason for your absence.

When is an RSVP unnecessary?

Invitations without an RSVP do not require them. For many of these events, the invitation may indicate "regrets only" as a way of getting a head count. In this case, you respond only if you are *not* planning to attend. Otherwise, your attendance is expected.

Is it OK to rearrange the place cards at a table?

No. Sit where the host wanted you to sit.

What should I do if I end up with something in my mouth that I don't like or can't chew?

Transfer it to your cocktail napkin and then place the napkin in a trashcan or on a service tray for collecting used plates and glasses.

If you meet someone at a cocktail party and suggest having lunch, what is the appropriate follow-up?

Don't suggest lunch unless you mean it. Be sure to follow up with a phone call or note within a few days.

How much should I tip a bartender?

The usual is $1 per drink at the bar.

(?) When should a guest leave a cocktail party?

It is polite to leave at or before the ending time for the event.
Don't overstay your welcome. If you are having a good time,
keep track of the time. If the invitation said that the event
would last from 5 to 7 p.m., don't stay a minute after 7 p.m.

**(?) Should I stand up if the host stands to make a toast
to someone?**

Yes. However, the person being toasted should remain seated.

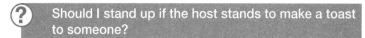

TAKE-AWAY TIPS

✓ Respond promptly to all invitations.

✓ Keep your conversation within appropriate
  parameters. Don't say anything to anyone
  that you will be embarrassed about later or
  that could get you into professional trouble.
  Remember, loose lips sink ships!

✓ Be discreet with your conversation. Avoid
  divulging your personal troubles.

✓ Avoid messy foods. Keep your hands clean
  for handshakes.

✓ You can be sociable and not drink alcohol.

✓ Business rules apply even in social settings.

✓ If in doubt, don't. For instance, if you
  question whether you should wear
  something, don't.

✓ If someone is toasting you, do not drink to
  yourself.

9

How Dining Etiquette and Business Success Go Hand in Hand

Seeing Through That Silverware Glare

Do you:

Know which water glass is yours?

Know what to do if you drop your fork on the floor?

Know which fork to use first?

Know what to do if you need to blow your nose at a meal?

Know what to do if someone asks you a question and your mouth is full?

These are concerns that can make you feel flustered or uncomfortable during a meal. The fast-food world and the school cafeteria do not provide many opportunities for learning the finer points of dining etiquette. However, minding your manners can make a lasting impression in a business or formal setting. Read on for guidelines to make you feel more comfortable and confident while dining during business meetings, job interviews, wedding receptions, and other special occasions.

Place Settings and Dining Utensils

Where is my bread plate?

One of the challenges of dining with others is figuring out which bread plate belongs to you and which water glass is yours. Fortunately, several mnemonic devices can make it easy to remember your way around a formal dinner table.

- All food to the left of the entrée plate belongs to you. This includes your salad, bread, and soup. An easy way to remember this is to note that *food* and *left* both have four letters.

- All drinks to the right of the entrée plate are yours. This includes your water, wine, and coffee cup. An easy way to remember this is to note that *drink* and *right* both have five letters.

- If you can remember the expression "leftover bread," you will be able to remember that your bread is on the left.

- Place the tip of your right thumb and forefinger together to make a circle. Straighten your fingers, and your hand will form a small letter *d*. Do the same with your left hand, and it will look like a small letter *b*. The *d* stands for *drinks* and indicates that your drink glasses (water, wine, and coffee) are on the right of your entrée plate. The *b* stands for *bread* and indicates that your bread plate is to the left of your plate.

- Another easy way is remember proper table setting positioning is to think of a BMW automobile. Here, instead of standing for *Bavarian Motor Works*, BMW stands for *bread*, *meal*, and *water*. Your bread is on the left, your meal is in the center, and your water glass is on the right. (Pagana, K. D., 2005a; Pagana, K. D., 2006b)

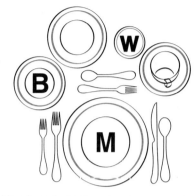

Your bread, meal, and water appear in this order from left to right, just like the letters of a BMW automobile.

✗ Faux Pas

As an acknowledgement of her Award for Clinical Excellence, Lindsey was being honored at a banquet attended by the medical center administration. She was so overwhelmed and confused by the many pieces of silverware, china, and glasses that she could not enjoy the meal or the conversation. She worried the entire time about making an etiquette blunder and leaving a bad impression on the administrators.

Which fork should I use first?

When it comes to dining utensils, a good rule of thumb is to work from outside to inside. The salad fork will be the smaller fork on the outside, and the larger dinner fork will be on the inside. Note that used utensils do not go back on the tablecloth. They are placed on the salad or entrée plate.

✗ Faux Pas

Mike had just finished his master's degree. He was invited to a business lunch as part of the interview process. Mike overheard the person to his right asking the waitstaff for a fork. He realized then that he was using the fork belonging to that person. He was embarrassed and worried about other etiquette blunders he may have committed.

What is the typical place setting for a four-course meal?

There are usually two forks to the left of the plate, two knives to the right of the plate, and a soup spoon to the right of the plate. (The smaller forks and knives are on the outside.) The soup spoon indicates that soup will be served first. After the soup spoon is removed, continue working from the outside in. The smaller fork and knife on the outside indicate that salad is the next course. After the salad, the larger fork and knife are used for the main course. The spoon and fork at the top of the place setting are for dessert.

When setting the table, which utensils go to the right and which go to the left of the entrée plate?

Here are a couple of tips to help you:

- The fork is placed to the left of the plate. *Fork* has four letters and so does *left*.

- The knife and spoon are placed to the right of the plate. *Knife* and *spoon* have five letters and so does *right*.

- Think of the mnemonic *FOrKS*. The *O* represents your circular entrée plate. The *F* stands for *forks*, which are placed to the left of the plate. The *r* indicates that the knives (*K*) and spoons (*S*) are placed, in that order, to the right (Post, 2014).

When setting the table, does it matter which way the blade of the knife is pointing?

Yes. Place the sharp edge facing the entrée plate.

Where do I put the napkin?

When everyone sits down at the table, napkins are placed on the lap. If you need to excuse yourself during the meal, place the napkin on your chair so others do not see your soiled napkin on the table. When the meal is finished and everyone is leaving the table, put the napkin to the left of the plate. If the plate is already removed, put the napkin where the plate was (Pagana, K. D., 2006c).

A waiter recently asked me if I wanted a black napkin. What was this about?

This is a nice gesture. Most restaurants set their tables with white napkins. Unfortunately, white napkins can leave white lint on dark clothing. Therefore, many restaurants also stock black napkins. If you see other patrons with black napkins, you can request one if you are wearing dark or black clothing. Often, in this situation, the waiter will ask you if you prefer a black napkin before you request one.

Bread and Butter

Who should pass the bread around?

If the bread is in a basket in front of you, pick it up and offer it to the person to your left. Then, take a piece yourself and pass it to your right. Or, you can just pick it up and pass it to your right (counterclockwise).

If someone already started passing the bread the wrong way, just go with it. Also, remember, as soon as you touch a piece of bread, it is yours. Do not reach into the basket and feel around for a hot roll on the bottom.

TIP

Do not serve yourself first.

How much bread can I butter?

If the butter is being passed around, put a pat of butter on your bread plate. When eating the bread, tear off a piece. Then butter and eat one piece at a time.

Some restaurants feature special oil for bread. If so, pour or spoon out a small amount onto your bread plate. *Never* dip your bread into the community oil.

What is the proper etiquette for handing a loaf of bread rather than individual pieces?

Let's start with what not to do. Do not pick up the bread with your bare hands and tear off a piece. Do use a cloth or napkin to hold the bread while you cut a few pieces with a knife. If you are served the bread without the cloth and knife, ask the waiter to bring them.

Soup and Salad

How do I handle the soup?

Many meals start with soup, which can be a challenge. Keep these points in mind:

- When eating soup, dip the spoon sideways into the soup toward the back of the bowl—that is, away from you. This technique prevents the soup from splashing onto your clothes.

- Skim the top of the soup with the spoon and sip from the side of your spoon, not from the front.

- Don't crumble crackers into the soup. Take one bite at a time, just like with bread.

- You can tilt the bowl away from you to get the soup from the bottom of the bowl. If the soup bowl has two handles, you can pick it up and drink from the bowl. However, this method is not widely known or commonly done.

- If the soup is hot, don't blow on it. Just wait until it cools down a bit. When you are finished, place your spoon next to the bowl on the plate. If there is no plate, leave the spoon in the bowl.

If the meal is during an important work meeting, it's best to avoid soups that are messy and hard to eat. Even if you love French onion soup, don't order it at a business meal. If it is pre-ordered, use your spoon to break the cheese against the back of the bowl so you do not stretch strings of cheese from the bowl to your mouth.

At a dinner party, one should eat wisely but not too well, and talk well but not too wisely.

—W. Somerset Maugham

Can I cut the salad?

Sure you can. Most salads do not have bite-sized pieces of lettuce. Therefore, use your knife and fork to cut the salad. Also, keep these points in mind:

- Be careful handling cherry tomatoes. Use one of the tines of your fork to poke into the stem area of the tomato. This will prevent the cherry tomato from shooting across the table when you cut it.

- If your salad has olives with seeds, use your fork to remove the seeds from your mouth and place them on the edge of your salad plate.

- If the salad dressing is in front of you, pick it up, offer it to the person on your left, serve yourself, and pass it to your right. Or, just pick it up and pass it to your right. The idea is not to serve yourself first.

Why should diners pass food to the right?

It simplifies dining when food is passed in one direction. Also, because most diners are right-handed, they receive the plate, basket, or salad dressing with their left hand, which leaves the right hand free to serve the food.

The Main Course

How many pieces of meat may I cut at a time?

This answer depends on whether you follow the American or Continental (sometimes called the European) style of dining. Although both are acceptable in the United States, the American style is most commonly used. The Continental style is the norm outside of the United States.

With the American style, sometimes called the *zig-zag style*, meat is cut with the knife in the right hand and the fork in the left. (The opposite hands are used for a left-handed person.) Two or three pieces of meat are cut at a time. Then, the fork is switched to the right hand to eat the meat. The knife is placed across the top of the plate with the blades pointing inward.

With the Continental style, the knife is again placed in the right hand and the fork in the left hand. With this style, however, each piece of meat is consumed as it is cut. The silverware is not switched to the other hand.

Table Manners Dos and Don'ts

Do:

- Say "please" and "thank you."
- Chew with your mouth closed.
- Pass the salt and pepper together.
- Place the salt and pepper shakers on the table in front of the person requesting them.
- Taste your food before seasoning.
- Wait for others to be served before starting to eat.
- Encourage others to start eating if your food is held up.
- Say "excuse me" if you have to go to the restroom during dinner.

Don't:

- Put your elbows on the table.
- Rearrange the place cards on the table.
- Wave your utensils.
- Slurp your soup.
- Pick your teeth.
- Blow your nose on the dinner napkin.
- Put on lipstick or makeup.
- Comb your hair.
- Ask for a doggie bag at a business meal or buffet.
- Say, "I have to go to the bathroom."

✗ Faux Pas

Several co-workers were eating dinner at an upscale restaurant in Philadelphia. One man pulled out some dental floss and flossed his teeth at the table. This uncouth behavior ruined the appetites of everyone else at the table. Although this behavior may be acceptable in other areas of the world, it is not appropriate in Pennsylvania.

Do you have any tips for fast eaters?

If you notice that you are likely to finish your meal well before everyone else, you must slow down your eating. Here are some tips to slow down your eating:

- Put your utensils down while chewing your food.

- Take smaller bites.

- Engage more in conversation.

Tips for Buffets

- Wait for the serving staff or host to direct your table to the buffet.

- Don't overload your plate. You can always go back after everyone has gotten food.

- Don't leave the serving spoon or fork in the serving dish. Place it on the saucer in front of the serving dish. This will prevent the handle from sliding into the serving dish.

- If you are the first one back to the table with food, wait for at least one other person to join you before you start to eat.

- Use a new plate when you return to the buffet.

- Don't ask for a doggie bag.

Do you have any tips for slow eaters?

It is important to keep pace with others at the table. If you are a slow eater, you need to pick up the pace. Here are some tips:

- While chewing your food, cut up food for the next bite.

- Take or order small servings.

- Answer questions in short sentences.

- Ask questions and eat while others talk.

Do you have any recommendations for handling difficult foods in a formal setting?

Yes. Don't order them at a formal setting. Save them for eating at home or with friends in an informal setting. Remember, this is not your "last supper"! Here are some tips for some challenging foods (Pagana, K. D., 2006b):

- **Bacon:** Generally, you should use a fork. However, if the bacon is crisp, you may pick it up with your fingers.

- **Bananas:** Peel the banana, cut into slices, and eat it with a fork.

- **Cherries with pits:** Use a spoon to put the cherry into your mouth and to remove the pit from your mouth.

- **Corn on the cob:** Butter a few rows at a time. When you eat it, hold it with both hands.

- **French fries:** Cut them into bite-sized pieces and eat them with a fork.

- **Lemons:** Cup the lemon in your hand to avoid squirting as you squeeze it over food or into drinks.

- **Parfait:** Start at the top and work your way down.

- **Pasta:** Use your fork to twirl a few strands against the edge of your plate.

- **Petits fours:** These are finger foods that are eaten in small bites.

- **Pork chops:** Use a knife and fork.

- **Cherry tomatoes:** Use the tine of the fork to poke into the area where the stem was attached. Then cut the tomato into pieces.

- **Watermelon:** Use a knife and fork. Use a spoon if the watermelon is shaped into small balls.

✘ Faux Pas

Barb and her husband went out to dinner with a work colleague, Denise, and her husband. While Barb was squeezing a lemon, the juice squirted across the table into Denise's eyes. The discomfort was significant for Denise, and it was several minutes before the group could continue the meal. Barb was mortified. After that, she wasted no time in learning how to handle difficult meal situations such as squeezing lemons.

Is there a way to signal to the waitstaff when I am finished with my plate?

Yes. You signal the waitstaff by positioning your silverware on your plate in the finished, rather than resting, position. The finished position signals to the waitstaff that the plate can be removed (Pagana, K. D., 2006a). In contrast, the resting position enables you to slow down and keep your plate on the table. This is particularly useful if you are a fast eater. Removal of your plate from the table puts pressure on others to speed up.

So what is the finished position and what is the resting position? The answer to that depends on whether you use the American style or the Continental style of dining. If you use the American style, imagine a clock on your plate. To indicate that you are resting and do not want your plate removed, place the fork with its top pointed at 10 o'clock and the base at the 4 o'clock position. The knife is placed across the top of the plate with the blade pointed inward. To indicate that you are finished, place the knife and fork in the 10 and 4 o'clock position with the tops of the silverware pointed at 10 and the bottoms pointed at 4.

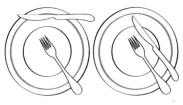

American: Rest   American: Finish

To indicate a resting position in the Continental style, place the fork and knife in an inverted V position. To indicate that you are finished, place the knife and fork in the 10 and 4 o'clock position with the tops of the silverware pointed at 10 and the bottoms pointed at 4. (This is the same as the American style.)

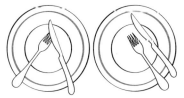

Continental: Rest   Continental: Finish

✗ Faux Pas

In her new position as vice president of nursing, Veronica was invited to a corporate dinner at an exclusive private dining club with the members of the board of trustees. She was served an exquisite meal by a doting waitstaff. During the meal, she was asked a question, and she put her silverware on her plate. With an attentive waitstaff, someone was there in a flash to whisk away her plate. Unfortunately, Veronica had placed her silverware in the finish position. She was stunned, and her facial expression gave away her surprise to her dinner partner, who was gracious enough to discreetly alert Veronica to the importance of handling silverware appropriately during a formal dinner. Veronica decided then and there to learn as much about dining etiquette as she could before the next dinner party.

Paying the Bill

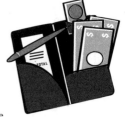

Who pays the bill?

The host should pay the bill and leave the tip. (Be prepared, however, in case the host does not know this.) The host should be able to figure out the tip without using a calculator. Good service usually is acknowledged with an 18 to 20% tip. Apps are available for quick tip calculations.

✓ Good Idea!

Amy was planning to take her father and stepmother out for dinner to celebrate her father's birthday. Two days before the dinner, she called to verify the reservation. While on the phone, she found out that the restaurant accepted only cash as payment. She had been unaware of this policy prior to calling to confirm the reservation and would not have had the necessary cash. Amy now asks about payment policies when she makes reservations.

X Faux Pas

Colleen and four of her co-workers were invited to dinner by their manager to celebrate the completion of a successful project. Colleen ordered a soup and salad. The manager ordered prime rib. When the waiter gave the bill to the manager, he divided it by six and told everyone to pay an equal share of the bill. The manager's inconsiderate decision was very upsetting for Colleen, because she only ordered what she knew she could afford. Because the manager invited Colleen and her co-workers out to dinner, he should have paid the bill.

What if the group ends up paying separately?

If everyone will be paying separately, alert the server before ordering to let him or her know to provide separate checks. For a shared check, be sure to have cash on hand to pay for everything you ordered, including tax and tip. If everyone ordered the same thing, divide the check after adding the tip.

✓ *Good Idea!*

In her position as vice president, Candace often hosts meals for male and female colleagues. To avoid an uncomfortable moment when the dinner check arrives, Candace gives the maître d' her credit card ahead of time and asks to have a 20% tip added. After the meal, she is presented the bill and merely has to sign it. She tells everyone that they are guests of the organization.

🌍 International Considerations

What are some considerations for dining in other countries?

When dining in other countries, you must consider many differences. These include the following:

- Where to sit at the table

- Where to place your hands during the meal

- How to signal when you've had enough food

See Chapter 12, "Going Global," for details and examples.

Are there differences in tipping?

Yes. Outside the United States, the tip is usually included in the bill. If the service was good, you can leave a little extra. Research the tipping practices of the country you are planning to visit beforehand.

Frequently Asked Questions

 Where should women place their purses when dining?

If the purse is small, it can go on the person's lap, under the napkin. If it's a large purse, she should put it on the floor between her feet or by her right foot, with the plan to exit the seat by the right side. Purses should not be placed on the backs of chairs. They can be in the way of the servers and also get stolen easily.

 How do I let the waiter know when I am ready to order?

Close your menu when you are ready to order. You can also catch the waiter's eye and nod your head indicating that you are ready.

 Should I turn over my coffee cup to indicate that I do not want coffee?

No, never turn over any plate, cup, or wine glass.

 What do I do when the silverware at the restaurant is wrapped in the napkin?

Carefully unwrap the napkin so you don't drop the silverware on the floor. Then place the silverware where it belongs in the place setting. Forks go to the left of the plate and knives and spoons to the right. Put the napkin on your lap.

 May I tuck the napkin into my collar?

No. However, you may lift your napkin up and cover your shirt for a few seconds when eating something messy. Men should not swing their tie around the back of their neck.

What foods should *not* be ordered at a business meal?

Avoid anything you do not know how to eat and anything messy. Examples of messy foods include spaghetti, barbecue ribs, and French onion soup. Eat messy foods on your own time and with your family and friends. Also, don't order expensive food like lobster or steak unless the host encourages you.

Before going to a business meal at an unfamiliar restaurant, is it a good idea to get some information about the restaurant?

Yes. This would be helpful. You could do this online. You would be able to see the menu and learn about specialty dishes. You might also learn some local history about the place that would make for interesting conversation.

May I dip my bread into the sauce on my plate?

Tear off a piece of bread and put it on your plate. Use your fork to spear the bread, dip it into the sauce, and eat it.

Before passing the salt to someone across the table, it is OK to salt my food?

No. Pass the salt and pepper as a pair to the requester. Then, politely ask to have the salt passed to you. Both salt and pepper should be passed together to you.

May I ask for an extra condiment, such as ketchup, steak sauce, or dressing?

Yes. Don't keep others waiting, however. Encourage them to start eating.

What if I have food in my mouth when someone asks me a question?

Point to your mouth and the questioner will get the hint. To take the pressure off you, he or she should ask someone else a question so everyone isn't looking at you and waiting for you to answer the question.

 What should I do if I get a fish bone in my mouth?

Use your fingers to remove the fish bone. Place it on the edge of your plate.

 How do I get a piece of meat gristle out of my mouth?

Most etiquette experts advise removing something from your mouth with the same utensils used to put it into your mouth. In this case, that would mean using your fork. However, many people do not feel comfortable doing this and remove the meat with one hand while using the napkin to block their mouth and dab their face with the other hand. Place the meat on the rim of your plate, preferably under a piece of garnish.

 Should I tell a dinner partner if he or she has poppy seeds in his or her teeth?

Yes. People want to know this.

 Are there any conversational topics to avoid during a meal?

Yes! Avoid discussing religion, politics, health problems, and anything inappropriate. If someone raises one of these topics in conversation with you, change the subject. For example, say, "How are your plans coming along for your anniversary cruise?"

What should I do if I drop my fork under the table?

Leave it there so you are not disappearing under the table during the meal. Ask the waitstaff for another fork.

What should I do if the server asks me to keep my knife when the table is being cleared?

You have two options here. One is to place your knife on your bread plate. (Never put a used utensil back on the table). The other is request a clean knife for the next course (Post, 2014).

Is it polite for the meal guest to offer to pay the tip?

No. This is because the guest would have to know the cost of the meal to calculate the tip.

If I am expecting an important call or text message, is it OK to check my cell phone during dinner?

You would need to have a compelling reason to do this. If you do, inform the host of this possibility and reason before the meal. If you receive a message or call, excuse yourself from the table to handle the disruption.

TAKE-AWAY TIPS

✓ If you are trying to decide how much you can spend on your meal, ask your host for food recommendations. If the host says he or she will be getting filet mignon, you can feel free to order it also. Without any recommendations or suggestions, stay in the middle price range.

✓ When you sit at the table, enter your seat from the left and exit from the right. This is especially important at a round table when 8 or 10 people are entering and exiting their chairs.

✓ Food is delivered to the table on your left side and removed from your right side. An easy way to remember this is the two Rs: *remove* from the *right.*

✓ Pass all food to the right. It is easier if food is going in one direction.

✓ Leave the table if you need to blow your nose.

✓ Don't chew gum at the table.

✓ When unsure of how to handle a certain type of food, sit back and watch others.

✓ Follow the lead of the host. If he or she passes on dessert or coffee, you should, too.

✓ A business meal should focus on business more than food. Remember, this is not your "last supper."

✓ When eating with international visitors, be respectful of different eating habits.

10

Thank-You Notes and Business Letters

How Expressing Yourself Can Make an Impact

Do you:

Wonder if it is proper to send a thank-you note by email?

Know the proper way to format a business letter?

Know thank-you notes are important but wonder when to send them?

Know the recipient's title, how to spell his or her name, and so on?

Know to whom the letter should be addressed?

Your written words are going to leave an impression. Your challenge is to make this a positive impression, because the written word has permanence and creates a paper trail. Many people are great communicators in face-to-face contact, but they are befuddled when they have to write a letter or note.

✓ Good Idea!

Recently a nursing assistant received Christmas gifts for her children from the nursing staff. In addition to thanking everyone profusely in person, the nursing assistant followed up with thank-you notes from her whole family. This meant a lot to the staff.

✗ Faux Pas

When her son graduated from high school, Eileen had a big party for him. A week after the party, the guests received a typed thank-you note addressed to family, neighbors, and friends. It was unsigned and the names on the envelope were written in Eileen's handwriting. It was obvious that Eileen had done everything. She missed an important opportunity to teach her son good manners.

Thank-You Notes

If I thank someone for something, is it really necessary to also send a thank-you note?

Yes. If you want to demonstrate good manners, show appreciation, and be remembered, send a thank-you note. A thank-you note is the 5-minute difference between feeling grateful and showing your gratitude (Spade, 2004).

Gratitude is the most exquisite form of courtesy.

—Jacques Maritain

Is it OK to email a thank-you note for a gift?

Only if you are following it with a note. If you are thanking someone for a gift or an event, send a handwritten note. Two or three sentences are all that is needed. Make sure you refer to the gift or the event. Emails do not have the same impact because they require only a few seconds of time and effort.

✓ Good Idea!

Three different administrators interviewed Jacqueline for a new position. During each interview, Jacqueline noted how each person's office was decorated. One office had golf photos, another had small statues of frogs, and the third had pictures of flowers. After the interview, she went to the mall and got thank-you cards featuring golfers, frogs, and flowers. She got the competitive edge by tailoring the cards to fit the personalities of the interviewers.

What about sending a note after an interview?

You have some options here. If you are sending a note after an interview, the note can be handwritten or typed, depending on its length. If you want to write more than several sentences, two typed paragraphs are acceptable. Try to mention one thing you had in common with the interviewer—for example, you both worked in New York earlier in your careers.

Thank-you notes received after interviews are usually placed in the applicant's file. When the applicants are reviewed, a note on nice paper will reflect better on your manners than an email.

TIP

At work, many people tack a thank-you note on a corkboard.

That being said, email is now another option for sending a thank-you note after an interview. In fact, some job candidates are now told to limit all follow-up correspondence to email. This is for the convenience of the interviewer and to give him or her the ability to quickly respond to questions or concerns.

When should I send a thank-you note?

All etiquette books agree that the sooner the better. For maximum impact, send the note as soon as possible after receiving a gift or attending an event.

An engraved or printed thank-you card, no matter how attractive its design, cannot take the place of a personally written message of thanks.

–Emily Post

TIP

If you type a thank-you note, be sure to sign your name.

✓ Good Idea!

Mark had four interviews scheduled the week before his graduation. Before the interviews, he purchased some fine quality thank-you cards. After each interview, he requested a business card. He wrote his thank-you cards in the evening after each interview and mailed them the next day. He made a good impression and had no trouble getting a position.

What if I forget to send a thank-you note and remember several weeks later?

Send the note. It is better late than never.

Examples of Thank-You Notes

Dear Theresa,

We had a wonderful time at your dinner party. The food was delicious and the company was most enjoyable. Thanks for inviting us.

> Sincerely,
> Jocelyn & Justin Balon

Dear Denise,

Christine and I enjoyed the holiday dinner party at your home. It was fun to be with so many nice people and share a delicious meal. Thank you very much.

> Happy Holidays!
> Ryan Flanery

Thank-You Note Etiquette Tips

- If you receive a gift or check, do not use the gift or cash the check until after you write the thank-you note.

- Thank the person for the specific gift and mention the gift by name. If the gift was money, don't mention the amount in your note. It is sufficient to say "your generous gift."

- Tell the person how the gift was or will be used.

- Send a thank-you note within a few days of receiving a gift or attending an event. If possible, do it within 24 hours.

- If you forget to send a thank-you note, go ahead and send it, even if it is several months late.

- Keep quality note cards and stamps on hand for writing thank-you notes.

 Do you have any suggestions for sending thank-you notes internationally after receiving a gift or having a phone interview?

Yes. Here are a few tips:

- Send the note as soon as possible after the interview, event, gift, or visit.

- Use quality stationery.

- Type or print the letter to avoid mistranslation due to handwriting idiosyncrasies. Although it is attractive, handwriting flourishes can be confusing for someone for whom English is a second or third language.

- Make sure you have the correct spelling of the person's name, and include his or her title. Check correspondence you have received from the person to verify this information.

- Print or type the address in the proper format for the designated country.

- Take the letter to the post office so it can be mailed with the proper postage and airmail designation.

Business Letters

Are business letters being replaced by email?

Today it is common to see business letters sent as email attachments. For example, contracts, purchase orders, and employment letters are usually sent by email with electronic signatures.

What are the key components of a business letter?

Business letters should have the following components:

- Date
- Titles
- Addresses of sender and recipient

- Salutation
- Body or content
- Closing
- Signature

The body of the letter should be clear and succinct, with a focus on "what's in it for them." Here are some helpful tips (Post, 2014):

- Be clear in your thought process. Avoid jargon.

- Use active voice. For example, write, "Justin will contact the job candidate" rather than "The job candidate will be contacted by Justin." Active voice adds strength and brevity to your sentence structure.

- Avoid using run-on or incomplete sentences.

- Vary the sentence structure.

- Use paragraphs. Paragraphs should be composed of 2 sentences at a minimum, but not more than 4 or 5 sentences or about 7 to 9 lines. Double space between paragraphs for easier reading.

- End your message. For example, say "I look forward to meeting you." Or, "Thank you for your time and consideration."

- Use a complimentary close, such as "Sincerely," "Sincerely yours," "Best regards," or "Cordially."

- If you are enclosing materials with your letter, type "Enclosure," "enc," or "encl."

- If you are distributing your letter to others, indicate courtesy copies by typing "cc" or "copies to." The names of the recipients should then be listed alphabetically.

What are some common mistakes with business letters?

Table 10.1 lists some common mistakes with business letters and tips on how to avoid making them.

 Common Mistakes with Business Letters

Mistake	*Tip*
Misspelling the recipient's name or title	Call the secretary or check the website.
Having typos in the letter	Use spell check and have someone else proofread your letter.
Using an informal tone	Keep the tone formal, even if you know the recipient. Others on a committee may see the letter.

| Forgetting to sign your letter | Check to make sure you signed the letter. Otherwise, you look unprofessional and show a lack of attention to detail. |
| Forgetting an attachment | If you say you are including something, make sure you add it before sealing and sending the letter. |

What are some tips for minimizing frustration and rewriting?

Organize your thoughts before you begin writing. Decide what you want to say and what you want as the outcome of your communication. Write a rough draft.

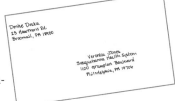

How can I avoid misspellings in a business letter?

Use your spell check. But remember, misspelled words can be overlooked by spell check when the misspelled word is a homonym—like *berth* and *birth*, *capitol* and *capital*, and *stationary* and *stationery*. A misspelled word can also be overlooked by spell check when the misspelled word is another real word—like *fist* instead of *first* or *bank* instead of *blank*.

Read your letter out loud. Have someone else read it for typos and misspellings. See the following list for some common misspellings in business letters.

Acceptance	Achievement	Anticipation
Approximately	Candidate	Commitment
Confidential	Conscious	Correspondence
Definitely	Equipped	Exceptionally
Fortunately	Immediately	Inconvenience
Irrelevant	Necessarily	Occasionally

Opportunities	Perceive	Perseverance
Philosophy	Possess	Practically
Receipt	Recommend	Schedule

Sample Business Letter

23 Hawthorn Road
Broomall, PA 18900
610-453-1993
Denise.Deska@denisedeska.com

April 15, 2015

Ms. Veronica Jones, MSN, RN
Vice President of Nursing
Susquehanna Health System
1100 Grampian Boulevard
Philadelphia, PA 14706

Dear Ms. Jones:

I saw your ad in *Pennsylvania Nurse,* and I would like to apply for the position of Clinical Practice Coordinator of the Oncology unit. I have just completed my MSN at the University of Pennsylvania with a clinical specialty in oncology. My BSN is from Lycoming College, and I have eight years' experience in medical-surgical nursing with the last four in oncology.

I have included a resume and a list of references with contact information. I would welcome the opportunity for an interview.

Thank you for your consideration.

Sincerely yours,

Denise K. Deska

Denise K. Deska, MSN, RN

Enclosures

How can I avoid errors with words with different meanings
that look alike or sound alike?

To avoid errors with words with different meanings that look alike
or sound alike, use your spell and grammar check. Also, have someone else proofread your letter. The following box contains common
errors.

Common Writing Traps

Affect and **effect**

- *Affect* is usually a verb, meaning to influence.
- *Effect* as a noun means result; as a verb, it means
  to bring to pass.

*The new legislation affected mandatory overtime, and
this effect supported nurse recruitment.*

Among and **between**

- *Among* introduces more than two items.
- *Between* introduces two items.

This honor should be shared among the entire staff.

This matter should be kept between the two of us.

Bring and **take**

- *Bring* indicates motion toward a person.
- *Take* indicates motion away.

Please bring this water to Mrs. Miller.

Take the dinner tray from the room.

Can and **may**

- *Can* implies ability.
- *May* implies permission.

Jerry may obtain the blood sugar if he can.

Complement and compliment

- *Complement* refers to something that completes.
- *Compliment* refers to praise.

The color of that scarf complements your suit.

He gave me a very nice compliment about my scarf.

Emigrate and immigrate

- People *emigrate* or move out of one country;
- They *immigrate* or move into another country.

The Irish emigrant was given permission to immigrate to the United States.

Farther and further

- *Farther* refers to a physical distance.
- *Further* means more or additional, and is used as a time or quantity word.

Move that desk farther to the right.

Let's take the point one step further to its logical conclusion.

Fewer and less

- *Fewer* refers to items that you can count.
- *Less* refers to degree or quantity.

There are fewer nurses in the same day surgery unit, and they have less experience than the recovery room nurses.

Irregardless and regardless

- *Irregardless* is not a word and should not be used.
- *Regardless* means despite or in spite of something.

The budget has been predetermined, regardless of what transpires in the meeting.

Me and I

- *Me* is the object of a verb or preposition.
- *I* is the subject of a sentence.

This problem is between you and me.

I am certain this is the correct route.

Stationary and stationery

- *Stationary* means fixed in place.
- *Stationery* refers to writing materials.

Once correctly installed, the new digital mammography machine remained stationary.

I will write my thank-you notes using my new stationery.

Was and were

- *Was* is used for things in the past. (Use *were* if the subject is plural or *you*.)
- *Were* expresses a wish or states a doubtful situation.

I was surprised to find you there.

If I were a college student today, I would choose nursing as a career.

Who and whom

- *Who* is used for the person who is the subject of a sentence.
- *Whom* (the objective case of who) refers to the person who has been the object of an action.

Who brought the new equipment?

The new equipment is to be used for whom?

Is a shorter letter more professional than a longer letter?

Yes. Be clear and concise. Don't waste the reader's time with un-necessary information. Read what you have written and eliminate any extra words or data. For guidance, see *The Elements of Style*, the classic grammar book written by William Strunk, Jr., and E. B. White. This little book is often described as the best primer on writing. It provides more information in less space than almost any other book.

> Do not be tempted by a twenty-dollar word when there is a ten-center handy, ready, and able.
>
> –William Strunk, Jr., and E. B. White

TIP

Edit, edit, edit. Eliminate grammar problems, spelling errors, and poor style.

How should I handle the address and salutation of a letter if I do not know the sex of the recipient?

Try to Google the person. If you are unsuccessful, drop the courtesy title in the address and salutation to avoid risking an unintended insult. For ex-ample, use "Pat Stanley" and "Dear Pat Stanley."

What should I write when I am addressing a position rather than a specific person?

Address the position, such as, "Dear Infection Control Nurse." This is preferred over "To whom it may concern." Or, a better way to handle this might be to call the organization and get the person's name. Often, when people receive communications that are not addressed to them by name, they assume they are marketing materials and toss them out.

Are there any particular phrases that should be avoided when writing?

Yes. See Table 10.2 for some windbag phrases and their substitutions.

10.2	Windbag Phrases

Windbag Phrases	Concise Replacements
Due to the fact that	Because
The reason why is that	Because
As per your request, enclosed please find	I have enclosed
Enclosed herewith	Here is
Until such time	When
As to when	When
In connection with	About
Subsequent to	After
As to how	How
Any and all	All
Prior to	Before

Brevity is the soul of wit.

—William Shakespeare

Memos

Has email replaced the office memo?

Although email has replaced many memos, the office memorandum, or *memo*, is still used for some interoffice correspondence. They are often attached to emails. Memos are generally used to transmit ideas, suggestions, or announcements. They provide a clear record of decisions made and actions taken.

What are the main components of a memo?

Most memos are formatted with four headings—*Date*, *To*, *From*, and *Subject*—followed by the body of the message. These headings can be in any order.

Be specific with the heading. For example, rather than saying "Isolation Protocol," use "Ebola Isolation Protocol." The heading also aids in filing and retrieval.

The body of the memo is similar to the body of a letter. Double space between the four headings and triple space between the last heading and the first paragraph of the memo. Limit the memo to one topic or message.

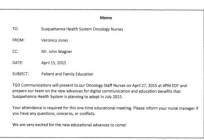

Memo

TO:	Susquehanna Health System Oncology Nurses
FROM:	Veronica Jones
CC:	Mr. John Wagner
DATE:	April 15, 2015
SUBJECT:	Patient and Family Education

TGD Communications will present to our Oncology Staff Nurses on April 27, 2015 at 4PM EDT and prepare our team on the new advances for digital communication and education benefits that Susquehanna Health System is planning to adopt in July 2015.

Your attendance is required for this one-time educational meeting. Please inform your nurse manager if you have any questions, concerns, or conflicts.

We are very excited for the new educational advances to come!

Is there a protocol for the To section?

There are several ways to handle this. It is best to follow the protocol of your organization. Here are some options:

- List the recipients of the memo in alphabetical order.

- List the recipients in descending order of corporate ranking. For example, the president's name should precede the chief financial officer.

- Mix the two systems. List one or two prominent names followed by an alphabetical listing of the remaining names.

- If the audience is a specific group, address the memo that way, without listing names —for example, To: The Breast Health Center.

Where is the memo signed?

There is no designated place for a signature on a memo. You can sign your name or initials after the From line or at the end of the memo.

Frequently Asked Questions

 Is it OK to send a thank you by email for a baby shower gift?

No. Sending a thank you by email should be an option only if you do not plan to send a handwritten note. Email is better than no mail, but it is always a second choice to a handwritten note, especially for a gift. An email does not convey the message that you went out of your way to send your thanks. It appears to be a hasty attempt to cross a task off your to-do list. However, it is OK to use email to thank a colleague for a small favor. This is different from receiving a gift or being taken out for dinner.

 Should I type a thank-you note if I have poor handwriting?

No. Neatly print a short note and sign your name. However, if your note is longer than a few sentences, type it.

Is there a proper way to fold a business letter before inserting it into an envelope?

Yes. A business letter is folded in thirds. First, fold the bottom third up. Then fold the top third down. Insert the letter into the envelope so it is right side up and readable when removed from the back of the envelope.

 How do I address a thank-you note to two people with different surnames who live at the same address?

Each person gets a line for his or her name. If it is a man and a woman, the woman's name is listed first.

 How do I address a letter or thank-you note to a couple where one or both are doctors?

Here are some options:

- Dr. and Mrs. Brian Myers

- Dr. Linda Myers and Mr. Brian Myers

- Doctors Brian and Linda Myers

- Dr. Linda Myers and Dr. Brian Myers

 Should I use a comma or a colon after the salutation line in a business letter?

The colon is preferred for most business letters (for example, Dear Ms. Dewar:).

TAKE-AWAY TIPS

✓ Think of a thank-you note as the 5-minute difference between feeling grateful and showing gratitude.

✓ Whenever someone gives you time, advice, a gift, or a helping hand, send a thank-you note.

✓ When it comes to business letters and memos, brief and to the point is far better than long and wordy.

✓ Neatness counts. Your letter is a stand-in for you.

✓ Err on the side of politeness. Use "Ms.," "Mrs.," or "Mr." until you have established a mutual rapport.

✓ Who doesn't enjoy receiving a thank-you note in the mail?

✓ Invest in good quality stationery for your business letters.

✓ Don't use a postage meter when sending thank-you notes. Use a stamp.

✓ A late thank-you note is better than no note at all.

✓ Bad grammar leaves a bad impression, especially with business letters and memos.

✓ Proper grammar and spelling demonstrate your care and attention to detail.

11

Jet Setting to Success

Business Travel and Etiquette

Do you:

Know the best way to get from the airport to your hotel?

Wonder if you should check your luggage or carry it on the plane?

Feel uncomfortable eating alone?

Feel concern for your safety?

Know how much to tip when traveling?

There is no doubt it: Business travel can be stressful, and stress makes it hard to demonstrate the kindness, consideration, and common sense associated with etiquette. Things do go wrong, and the unexpected does happen. However, if you know some basics, you will decrease your stress and increase your chance of having an enjoyable trip.

A good traveler focuses on three basic objectives:

- Being prepared

- Being self-reliant

- Being flexible

Read on to find out how to be a good traveler and bring your business etiquette along with you on your trip.

No act of kindness, no matter how small, is ever wasted.

—Aesop

Packing with Precision

What should I pack?

Carefully plan your packing. Pack only what you need and leave the rest at home. Mix and match outfits as much as possible.

Think of the events you will attend during your trip and plan your outfits for each one. I find it helpful to place my outfits with accessories out on my bed before putting them in my suitcase.

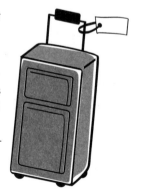

I use a travel checklist every time I pack. I cross off anything that does not apply to the trip and then check off everything else as I pack it. See the following boxes for suggestions on developing your own customized list.

Packing List for Personal Items

Program/Event
- Suit
- Shirt/extra shirt
- Shoes
- Stockings or socks
- Underwear
- Jewelry

Night Clothes
- Robe
- Slippers
- Pajamas/ nightgown

Fitness
- Swim cap, swim-suit, and goggles
- Gym shirt
- Gym pants or shorts
- Sneakers/running shoes
- Jacket for outside exercise
- Sunscreen

Personal Items
- Makeup kit
- Toiletries
- Shaving kit
- Curling iron
- Contact lenses
- Medications

Miscellaneous
- Cell phone
- Phone charger
- Sunglasses, reading glasses
- Hat
- Earplugs

Packing List for Business Items

Hardware Essentials

- Computer
- Computer power source
- Program loaded on computer
- Program backed up on flash drive
- Extension cord

Travel Documents

- Hotel reservations
- Travel directions
- Airline reservations
- Photo identification
- Passport
- Contact information

Presentation

- Presentation notes
- Printed copies of presentation (PowerPoint)
- Clean, unmarked copy of the handouts
- Program details

Miscellaneous

- Business cards
- Tablet
- Highlighter
- Calendar
- Writing utensils

X Faux Pas

Angelina was excited to be presenting at a prestigious nursing conference. Although she had submitted her handout months ago, when she arrived, it was not available for the participants. The problem could have easily been resolved if she had brought a clean copy of the handout or a jump drive containing the handout. Unfortunately, the conference personnel had to retype the handout at the last minute. Now Angelina packs to prevent this reoccurrence.

How should I organize my suitcase?

Fold small items and place them in reusable, sealable bags, such as Ziploc bags. That way, nothing will get wet and nothing will spill (Pagana, T. N., 2008). This is a great way to organize and group items. For example, put all underwear in one bag.

Fold and then roll each garment separately, and then tuck each one into a quart, gallon, or 2-gallon sealable plastic bag. This cuts down on wrinkling and allows you to quickly find your items. When rolling pants, start at the hem and roll up. When folding shirts and sweaters, fold a section on each side with the sleeves back, and then roll from the bottom up.

TIP

Have a cosmetic kit or shaving kit always packed and ready to go. Refill necessary items after each trip.

Should I bring an iron?

No. Most hotel rooms have an iron and ironing board in the closet. If not, the hotel staff can usually supply one. You can call ahead to verify this or check the hotel's website for a list of amenities. If you unpack your clothes and find they are wrinkled, try hanging them in the bathroom while you take a hot shower. The steam will usually remove the wrinkles.

X Faux Pas

When Tim's flight landed, it was raining—hard. He was relieved to retrieve his luggage. However, when he unpacked at his hotel, he discovered that all of his clothes were wet. Everything had to be cleaned. Because of this experience, he now packs his clothing inside a plastic dry-cleaning bag. It doesn't take up any room, and it keeps his clothes dry.

If you are traveling overseas, you probably won't have access to an iron. Also, you may need to bring an adapter for electrical items because of different electrical currents. As an example, you will not be able to use an American blow dryer in France without an adapter.

✗ Faux Pas

Marianne was traveling for business and stayed in a very nice hotel. After showering, she tried to dry her hair with the blow dryer, but it did not work. By the time she received a replacement, she had only 10 minutes to dry and style her hair. She had to rush out of her room to be on time for her meeting. Now, she locates and tries the blow dryer as soon as she checks in.

Air Travel

If I need to fly out of town for business, who is responsible for scheduling my airline reservations?

This will vary. Some companies will give you guidelines for making your reservations and expect you to do it. The guidelines may include a maximum ticket price and what airport to fly into. Other companies will have a travel department with which you must connect to make your reservations. Companies usually have an expectation that all tickets be booked at least a month before the event to get the best airfare possible.

Is it a good idea to stick with one air carrier?

If possible and financially prudent, yes. You often get better seats if you are a frequent flyer. In addition, frequent flyers with a lot of earned miles often can board before other passengers, get seats near the front of the plane, and, when upgrades are available, be offered first-class seats. Also, frequent flyers build up points and can earn free flights.

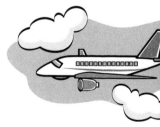

When my travel plans are finalized, who should get a copy of my itinerary?

The person you are meeting, your office, and your family should get copies. Make sure the itinerary includes the following essential details:

- The flight schedule, including the name of the airline, flight numbers, and departure and arrival times

- The name, address, and phone number of your hotel

- The locations and times of your meetings

- The name and contact information (including cell-phone number) of the person you are meeting

What can I do to prevent frustration with airplane delays and cancellations?

Prepare yourself by *not* expecting that everything will go well. Give yourself plenty of time to get to your destination. Never take the last plane of the day out of the airport. If it gets cancelled, you are really stuck. It is best to arrive much earlier than necessary to allow plenty of time to work or relax before business. Plan to arrive the day before any important event.

What should I do if my flight is cancelled?

This is an unfortunate situation, but handling it effectively is part of the flexibility needed to be a good traveler. Here are some suggestions:

- Do not get angry at the airline service personnel.

- While standing in line to speak to an agent, use your cell phone to call the airline or your travel agent to book another flight.

- Download the app for the airline to your smart phone. Use the app to find a new route to your destination.

- Ask the airline representative if any partner airlines can accommodate your travel.

- Inquire about meal tickets and hotel vouchers.

- Have important contact information with you and readily available. That way, if, for example, you are going to a job interview, you can notify the contact person about your situation.

What suggestions do you have to make my flight check-in go smoothly?

This is a stressful event for most travelers. Here are some suggestions:

- **Check the status of your flight beforehand:** Do this by phone or on the Web several hours before leaving your home for the airport. Print out your ticket within 24 hours of your departure time. You may be able to get a better seat at this time.

- **Bring photo identification:** Use your driver's license or passport.

- **Make sure your checked luggage does not exceed the weight restrictions:** This will be clearly stated on the airline's website. Hefty fees can result if you exceed the weight limit. Most airlines charge for luggage. However, if you are a frequent flyer with a lot of accrued miles, one or two bags may be free.

- **Make sure your carry-on luggage does not exceed the size limitations:** If you have two bags, put the larger one in the overhead compartment and the smaller one by your feet.

- **Check with the TSA on the policy for packing liquids:**
  Containers with more than a few ounces of liquid are
  not allowed in carry-on luggage. Your liquids, including
  toothpaste and creams, must fit into a 1-quart plastic bag.
  These policies are clearly described on airline websites and
  on the TSA website.

- **Arrive at the airport early:** Check the airline website or
  Transportation Security Administration website (www.tsa.
  gov) for suggested check-in times. Many airports advise
  arriving 1 to 2 hours before the flight time to get through
  security.

- **Arrive early for international flights:** For international
  flights, be at the airport at least 2 hours before the flight
  time. Be sure to bring your passport. Also, make sure you
  are in the right terminal. International departures from large
  airports, such as Chicago O'Hare or New York La Guardia,
  will often be in a separate terminal because of the larger
  aircraft.

- **Check the visa and entry requirements of each country
  before you book travel or depart:** For some destinations,
  such as Singapore, your passport must not expire less than 6
  months before your departure date.

- **Do not have any wrapped gifts in your carry-on luggage:**
  They may need to be unwrapped by TSA when your bag is
  scanned.

- **Eat before you leave home or bring some food:** Few airlines
  provide food or snacks on regular flights. In most cases,
  however, you can purchase a small meal or snack while in
  the air.

- **Do not leave your bags unattended or ask anyone to watch
  your bags:** This is a safety issue that is strictly enforced at
  airports.

Is it better to carry on my luggage or check it on the plane?

Both have advantages. If your trip is purely business, minimize your packing and carry on your luggage. If your trip is for pleasure, you can pack more things if you check your bag. However, make sure you carry any medications or valuables with you.

Plan for the possibility that your checked luggage will get lost or be delayed. Put some essentials—such as a toothbrush, toothpaste, and possibly a change of underwear—in your carry-on bag or purse.

Bring your manners with you on your trip.

How much do I tip the skycap at the airport?

The usual tip is $2 per bag. Some airports now charge a fee of $2 per bag, not including tip.

How should I dress on the plane?

This will depend on how soon you will be meeting people at your destination and whether you plan to check your bags. If you plan to meet people before you will have the opportunity to change, dress for that meeting. If you are checking your bags, wear something presentable in case your bags get lost. If you are carrying your bags and not meeting anyone until after you have checked in, you have more options for dressing in a casual manner.

Always carry a sweater or jacket. Wear slacks instead of shorts—even during the summer. You will be more comfortable in the airport and on the plane.

How can I demonstrate professional etiquette while flying?

Because flying can be stressful, and because you are in close quarters with many others, you need to demonstrate good manners. See the following box for some helpful tips.

TIP

Carry a small blanket with you. Blankets are no longer available on most flights unless you are in first-class seating.

Etiquette Tips for Flyers

- Wait your turn when boarding and disembarking from the plane.
- If you bring food onto the plane, make sure it does not have a strong odor.
- If your luggage does not fit in the overhead compartment or under the seat in front of you, tell the flight attendant so it can be checked.
- Ask your seatmate's permission before adjusting the window shades.
- Turn off your cell phone or keep it in airplane mode.
- Don't block the aisle for more than a few seconds when putting your luggage in the overhead compartment.
- Don't crush anyone's belongings in the overhead compartment to squeeze in your item.
- Don't ask to put your luggage in someone else's foot space.
- Keep your things in your own space.
- Don't stretch out into the aisle.
- Nod and say hello to your seatmates.

- Don't keep talking if the person next to you wants to sleep, work, or read.

- If the person next to you keeps talking and you don't feel like chatting, put on your earphones, open a book, or close your eyes for a nap.

- Don't try to read the computer screen of people nearby.

- If you are in the aisle seat and want to sleep, leave a way for others to get through without waking you up. For example, don't use the tray table as a headrest.

- Be courteous with the flight attendants.

- If the child sitting behind you is kicking your seat, talk to the parents instead of scolding the child. It's not appropriate to correct the behavior of someone else's child.

- Be considerate of the person seated behind you. If you want to recline your seat, it would be nice to warn the person whose space you are about to invade. In some planes, if you crank your seat back, you can end up in the lap of the person behind you. This is very annoying and prevents that person from working on his or her computer. Keep your seat up during meal times.

- When exiting the plane, let everyone ahead of you out first. Be ready to leave when it is your turn.

Rudeness is the weak man's imitation of strength.

--Lawrence Sterne

What are the options for transportation from the airport to the hotel?

Taxis are a convenient way to get to your hotel, especially if you are in a hurry and it is dark. Before traveling, call the hotel and ask for the usual fare from the airport to the hotel. It is also a good idea to use the Internet to get directions. You will find out the most direct route and the estimated time for travel. Carry small bills in case the driver cannot make change. Tip the driver 15 to 20% of the fare.

> **TIP**
>
> **Stand to the right and pass to the left on escalators or moving walkways in the airport.**

You can also hire a car service. In this case, you will have a car waiting for you and a person standing near the baggage claim area holding a sign with your name or company name. Because the cost is determined up front, there are no surprises. You can also pay with your credit card with most limousine services.

Other options for travel include trains, subways, and buses. Some hotels provide free pickup services. Find out about available services by calling the hotel ahead of time. If you are attending a conference, this information is usually available in the brochure or with the registration confirmation materials. Also, there are usually discounted shuttle rates for conferences. Shuttles can be booked online.

A new transportation option, similar to a taxi, is a service called Uber. With Uber, area residents provide transportation using their own cars. You can access this service by using the Uber app on a mobile device. Prices are set, and you can pay with a credit card. Tips are included in the price. Some people prefer this over the hassle of renting a car or the expense of taking a taxi.

Demonstrating Professional Etiquette on Trains, Subways, and Buses

As with airplanes, you are in close quarters with other travelers on these modes of transportation. Here are some tips:

- Board after everyone leaving has made it out the door.

- Minimize use of your cell phone. If you do have to use your cell phone, speak softly and briefly. Be aware that in some cases, cell phone use is prohibited. Don't distract others who are trying to read or relax.

- Don't spread out your things and tie up seats.

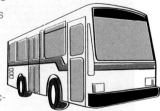

- Do offer your seat to pregnant, disabled, or elderly people.

- Be courteous to the conductor or driver.

Car Travel

What travel tips do you have for a road trip in my car?

You need to know exactly where you are going, how to get there, and how much time it takes. As with flying, don't make this a last-minute stressor. Here are some additional road-trip tips:

- Obtain the exact location of the event, including the zip code. This makes it easier to use a navigation system.

- Use an online mapping service, such as Google Maps, for directions.

- Print your directions in large type for easy reading.

- Rent or purchase a global positioning system (GPS) car navigator.

- Make sure your car is trip-ready. Fix any indicator alerts, such as a low oil level.

- Bring your sunglasses.

- Be aware of your gas level and keep it above a quarter of a tank.

- Travel with your cell phone.

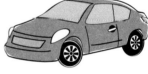

- Always lock your car doors.

- Park only in well-lit areas.

- If you feel uncomfortable, ask a security guard to walk you to your car.

- Leave only your ignition key with a parking attendant.

✓ Good Idea!

Monica was traveling across the country after attending a nursing symposium in California. Due to thunderstorms and air traffic delays, she arrived late in Philadelphia and missed the last commuter flight to her hometown. Her husband rented a car for her while she waited in a long line to retrieve her luggage. When she finally got to the car-rental site, it was 11:00 p.m., and the line for the counter extended out the door and around the corner. The estimated wait for a car was over one hour. She called her husband to give him an update. He told her that he already had paid for the car and to get into the Fast Track line. No one was in this line, and she had her car within 5 minutes! This tip has been invaluable in Monica's subsequent travels.

Do you have any recommendations for renting a car?

Renting a car should be part of your pre-trip planning. Otherwise, you could get to your destination and not be able to rent a car. Here are some tips:

- Have a copy of your rental-car reservation in your hand when you meet the agent.

- Be careful of the agent's push to sell unneeded services. Your own car insurance is usually enough, but be sure to check with your insurance agent if this is your first time renting a car.

- Do not agree to pay a cheaper gas price for the car-rental agency to fill the tank when you return the car unless you plan to return the car on empty. They will charge to fill the entire tank, even if you only needed a few gallons. Your best option is usually to fill the car yourself right before you return it to the rental agency and pay only for the gas you used.

- Do not discuss any private business on a cell phone or with a co-worker on the rental-car shuttle bus. You never know who is on the bus and how they might use your information.

- Check to make sure the gas tank is full before you leave the lot.

- Make sure you have directions before you leave the lot. You can get a map from the rental company. However, it is usually better to bring your own directions from a service such as Google Maps.

- Consider renting a GPS to avoid getting lost in an unfamiliar area.

- Try to pick up and return rental vehicles during daylight hours.

- Keep the car doors locked at all times.

- Put your luggage in the trunk.

Hotels

How can I stay safe when staying alone in a hotel?

This is an important issue, especially for women traveling alone. Following are some safety tips for when you stay in a hotel:

- Keep your room number private. If the bellman asks for your room number, show your key rather than say the number.

- If the desk clerk makes your room number public, ask for a different room.

- When shopping in the gift shop or eating in the dining room, don't mention your room number when you are charging something to your room.

- If it is dark and you are fearful, have the bellman enter your room with you and stay while you check the room.

- If you are uncomfortable about the location of your room, ask to have it changed. It's a good idea to ask for a room that is not on the ground floor when you make your reservation or when you are checking in.

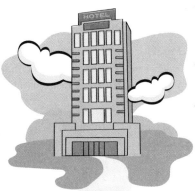

- Do not open the door if anyone knocks. Call the front desk to verify any room work or service.

- Bolt the door and apply the safety latch.

- If there is a sliding door, make sure it has a safety latch and a metal bar.

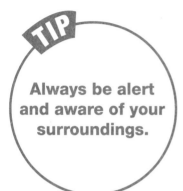

Always be alert and aware of your surroundings.

✓ Good Idea!

Elizabeth was traveling to speak at a conference. She got to her hotel early and checked in. When she got to her room, she found it was not part of the main hotel. It also did not have an inside entrance, and the room was on the ground floor. Not feeling safe, she returned to the registration desk to discuss her concerns. She was switched to a nicer room with a safer, inside entry. Safety is a number one concern for women traveling alone, and hotels will do their best to accommodate solo travelers.

- If your room has a connecting door, make sure it is locked. If possible, try to book a room without a connecting door. You can also request this at check-in.

- Don't leave the door open with the latch lock if you leave the room to get ice.

- Always have your room key out and ready to use as you walk to your room.

- Use the room safe to secure your valuables.

- Make sure your door closes and locks every time you leave the room.

- Keep a light on in the room when you leave so it is not dark when you return.

- If the hotel fitness center does not have an attendant and you feel unsafe, use the facility only when other people are around.

- Use valet parking if you arrive late. That way, you won't have to walk through a dark parking lot alone (Rickenbacher, 2004).

- If you are leaving your room after it has been cleaned, put out the "do not disturb" sign so it appears that someone is in the room.

If I need to hold a business meeting at the hotel, is it OK to use my hotel room?

No. Arrange to use a meeting room. Or, meet in a dining room. It is too personal to meet in your hotel room, especially when with a member of the opposite sex.

Should I bring an alarm clock?

This depends. Most hotels have alarm clocks. Check the alarm clock when you get into the room. (Note that the alarm may still be set by the previous person.) If you cannot figure out how to set the alarm, call the front desk. For some people, it is more convenient to bring a small travel alarm that they know is dependable and that they know how to use. I prefer to use the alarm on my cell phone.

Should I use the wake-up call service?

Yes. This is a great idea. However, have a backup strategy. Sometimes, the call system goes down. Also, be certain to hang up the phone properly after placing the call to schedule the service or it will not ring in the morning. Use the alarm in your room or on your cell phone as a backup.

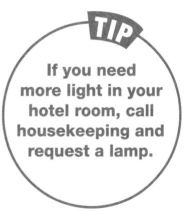

TIP

If you need more light in your hotel room, call housekeeping and request a lamp.

Do I need to bring my computer to a hotel?

It depends. Bring your computer if you need it for your work. Otherwise, many hotels have a business center with computers. In some cases, there is a small fee for usage. Call in advance to learn about computer and printer usage at your hotel.

Back up presentations on a flash drive or email them to yourself in case of technical difficulties. If you have emailed the presentation to yourself, you could use someone else's computer.

Is Internet service available in most hotels?

Yes. It is not always free, however. Often, the charge is about $10 to $15 per day. This is billed on a 24-hour period or billed as a full day until the next day's checkout time. Interestingly, low-cost hotels often have free Internet service.

If my conference lists several hotels, which one should I choose?

Find out which hotel is hosting the conference. That would be most convenient. Check other hotels for distance, price, and amenities. You may also be able to find another nearby hotel that was not listed but is available at a cheaper rate.

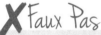

X Faux Pas

Kathy and her 78-year-old father were checking out of a hotel when Kathy saw her dad putting all the snack items in his suitcase. He thought the snack items were free. He did not realize that every snack or minibar item missing from the room would be charged to the room bill. These room items are also priced much higher than those in the gift shop.

How can I expedite checking out of a hotel?

You should receive a copy of your bill under your door on the morning of checkout. Review all of the charges and read the check-out instructions. In many cases, you can call a number and indicate the time when you are vacating the room. You may also be able to check out using the TV or a kiosk in the hotel lobby. If you are un-sure of any items on your bill, call or go to the front desk to discuss them. Everything will be charged to the credit card you have on file, and your balance should be $0 on your statement. Receipts can also be sent by email.

If I am sharing a hotel room, how can I get a receipt for my expenses?

This can easily be done at the front desk. The clerk can separate the charges and give both of you an individualized, itemized receipt.

Handling Expenses and Reimbursements on a Business Trip

Before you begin your trip, find out what will be reimbursed and what the caps are for reimbursement. For example, you may be limited to a per diem of $30, or a meal total of $30. You also may be reimbursed for a shuttle service, but not for a taxi.

Keep receipts for everything. It is very helpful if you have a designated place for keeping receipts. You will need an itemized hotel bill if you charged your meals to your room. Alcoholic beverages are not usually reimbursable. As soon as your return from your trip, make a copy of your receipts and submit your reimbursement form. Most companies have a time limit for submitting these forms. Often this limit varies from 3 to 30 days.

Are there etiquette guidelines for tipping in a hotel?

Yes. It is a good idea to travel with a lot of $1 bills for tipping. Here are some suggestions for tipping (Fox, 2007; Post, 2014):

- **Maid who cleans your room:** At least $2 per night

- **Doorman who carries your bag:** $2 for the first bag and $1 per additional bag

- **Bellman who carries your bags to your room:** $2 for the first bag and $1 per additional bag

- **Concierge who gives you a map and directions:** No tip

- **Concierge who makes dinner reservations for you:** $10 to $20

- **Concierge who finds hard-to-get theatre tickets for you:** $10 to $20 per ticket

- **Doorman who hails a cab:** $1

- **Waitstaff in a restaurant:** 15 to 20% of the tab (excluding tax)

- **Room service waitstaff:** No tip or $1 (the gratuity is usually added to the bill whenever you order room service)

- **Valet parking:** $1 to $2

Frequently Asked Questions

 Should I carry my blow dryer on a trip?

No. Most hotels have these in the room. Call the hotel to verify this.

 I am often asked to change seats on a plane so family members can sit together. Am I obligated to switch?

Not at all. The frustrating part of being asked to move is that you may have paid for an expensive aisle seat. The family who wasn't willing to pay more to get seats next to each other may now be making their thrift your problem. Do what you want and don't feel compelled to change seats (Post, 2014). Note, though, that sometimes flight attendants will provide seat upgrades or other amenities for you to move to accommodate families with small children.

❓ If I am traveling with a person of honor, who gets into the cab first?

You should get in first so you are the last out and can pay the driver. The person of honor should have the rear seat closest to the curb. This avoids the person needing to slide across the seat.

❓ How much should I tip a cab driver?

The usual tip is 15 to 20% of the fare on the meter. Add $1 per bag if the driver loads your bags in and out of the trunk.

❓ Is it OK to bring my spouse on a business trip?

Yes, if he or she knows that business comes first. Keep separate receipts for reimbursable expenses, such as meals.

❓ If I am traveling alone, should I order room service and eat in my room?

Not unless you want to. It is perfectly acceptable to eat by yourself in the dining room. It is common for travelers to eat alone. Bring a magazine or book to read until your food arrives. Many people check for messages on cell phones while they wait for their food.

TAKE-AWAY TIPS

✓ **Keep your travel clothing simple, lightweight, and wrinkle-free.**

✓ **Don't forget to pack clothes for evenings.**

✓ **If you do not know what to wear, ask your host.**

✓ **Carry a prescription for needed medications.**

✓ **Carry a lens prescription for glasses or contacts.**

✓ **Take inconveniences in stride.**

✓ **Maintain a confident but low-key profile.**

✓ **Make a copy of your itinerary and give it to a family member or friend.**

✓ **Have all luggage identified inside and outside.**

✓ **Before getting into a cab, confirm the fare.**

✓ **Trust your instincts. If you feel uncomfortable, leave.**

12

Going Global

Business and Etiquette Around the World

Do you:

Wonder how you should dress for business in another country?

Know if you should give a gift to your host?

Know that some gestures can be offensive, but don't know which ones to avoid?

Know handshaking etiquette for women?

Wonder how to present and receive a business card?

Know the dining etiquette differences in other countries?

As with all business travel, preparation, self-reliance, and flexibility are key components of a successful international travel experience. However, international travel and interactions are complicated by cultural differences in etiquette. Each culture has its own traditions, rules, and priorities. It is important to learn about these variations before setting out on your trip.

Important Note to Non-travelers

You may think you will not get any benefit out of reading this chapter. Wrong! As a healthcare professional, you interact with patients and providers from diverse cultural backgrounds. Reading this chapter will enhance your cultural awareness and sensitivity in your interactions with others.

Manners must adorn knowledge, and smooth its way through the world.

–Lord Chesterfield

Basic Preparations

What is an "ugly American," and how can I avoid being called one during my travels?

The term originated from the title of a 1958 book called *The Ugly American* by Eugene Burdick and William Lederer. The term describes Americans abroad who are perceived as arrogant, demeaning, and thoughtless. For example, you may come off as sounding superior and judgmental with comments such as, "I can't believe this restaurant does not have ice cubes" or "These people seem lazy, taking a siesta every day after lunch."

Educating yourself before you travel and having an appreciation for cultural differences can help you avoid this stigma. Remember, the American way is not the only way. Your behavior should not be offensive to the people whose country you are visiting.

What points of etiquette should I research as I make my travel plans?

What is polite and appropriate in one culture may be offensive in another. See the topics in the following box. Research these topics before you leave home. Use the Internet or get a guidebook. Or, see the resources listed near the end of the chapter.

TIP

Ignorance of business etiquette is simply not acceptable in the global arena.

Etiquette Research Prior to Travel

- Appropriate greetings
- Handshake, kissing, and bowing customs
- Public displays of affection
- Gift-giving etiquette
- Dress codes
- Gestures
- Eye contact
- Religious beliefs and customs
- Business interactions
- Social structure, such as the role of women in the culture
- The relationship between bosses and subordinates
- The concept of time (being prompt or late)
  (Pagana, K. D., 2013a; Purnell, 2012)

What are some basic facts I should learn about a country before my trip?

If you do your homework, you will avoid the lack of preparation that is a shortcoming for many U.S. travelers. The following list covers most of the basics to investigate so you can feel more comfortable and appreciate your travel adventures (Post, 2014):

- The correct name of the country (for example, the Czech Republic, not Czechoslovakia)

- The nation's capital

- The form of government

- The names of the top government officials

- Types of religion

- National holidays that occur during your trip

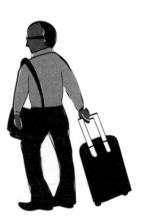

- Dietary laws

- Leading industries

- Type of currency and exchange rates

- Prominent geographical features (for example, Mount Kilimanjaro)

- Famous cultural landmarks (for example, the Catacombs)

- Famous men and women (for example, writers, musicians, and artists)

- Popular sports

Currency Conversions

To handle currency conversions, visit www.oanda.com. Then do the following:

1. Click the currency convertor.
2. Indicate the currency you have and the currency you want.
3. Click the Traveler's Cheatsheet option.
4. Print out this conversion table. You may want to tape it to a small index card.

This information is invaluable. With this information, you can estimate currency calculations without needing a calculator.

Should I try to speak the language in a foreign country?

Yes. Demonstrate your respect by learning a few words and key phrases. This information is free on the Internet. You can even find pronunciation guides. Even if you mispronounce the words, people will appreciate your effort. Here are some words to try to learn:

- Hello
- Goodbye
- Please
- Thank you
- Good morning
- Good afternoon
- Good night
- Excuse me

Carry a pocket dictionary or a list of phrases to help you communicate with people who do not speak English. Also, many language apps are readily available for mobile devices.

Do you have any suggestions for working with translators?

Yes. If you are using a translator to communicate with someone, look at and speak directly to the person instead of the translator. Avoid jokes. Humor does not translate well. You could easily offend someone.

How do I know how to dress for a business meeting while abroad?

This is definitely an area to investigate before packing. In general, dress on the conservative side until you see what your international colleagues are wearing. In most circumstances, women should avoid skirts or dresses above the knee. Women should be especially conservative in deeply religious countries. You should carefully investigate appropriate dress in these countries. A good place to begin your investigation is with the country link on the United States Department of State website (www.state.gov).

If I make an etiquette blunder, what should I do?

Your mistake may be obvious from someone's comments, expression, or body language. Apologize immediately. If you do not know what you did, say, "Please help me. Let me know what I did so I don't do it again." Demonstrate a humble and respectful attitude. It is not acceptable to simply say, "I didn't know."

If I am hosting a visitor from another country, how can I be a gracious host?

You can be a gracious host if you take time to learn about the person's culture. Here are some guidelines to ensure a nice visit (Pachter, 2013):

- Know the visitor's usual method of greeting.

- Learn about the visitor's customs and values.

- Meet or send someone to meet the person at the airport.

- Ask about dietary restrictions in advance, if possible.

- Send flowers or a basket of food to the person's room. Be culturally sensitive when making your selection.

- Arrange for transportation during the person's visit.

- Plan interesting things for the person to do.

- Invite the person to your home for dinner.

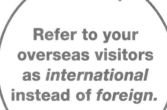

TIP

Refer to your overseas visitors as *international* instead of *foreign*.

Making Introductions

How should I greet an international business associate?

If you are not sure how to greet the person, start with a handshake or follow his or her lead. If the person greets you with a kiss, follow suit. You may offend the person if you pull away. A bow or a hug may be appropriate in other cultures.

How does handshake etiquette differ around the world?

In the United States, a firm handshake is used to communicate confidence and self-assurance. Don't judge people from other cultures by their handshakes. Here are some things to find out about handshakes (Pagana, K. D., 2013a):

- **Who initiates the handshake?** It may be the most senior person.

- **Do men wait for women to extend their hand?** Yes, in many European countries.

- **Can men shake a woman's hand?** Not if they are Muslim or Hindu.

- **Should the grip be gentle or firm?** In Denmark, Finland, Ireland, Norway, and Sweden, handshakes are firm but brief. In China, handshakes are softer and longer.

- **Is a bow the equivalent of a handshake?** Yes, in Japan and some other Asian countries.

If a bow is used instead of a handshake, who bows first?

In a rank-conscious society such as Japan, the person of lower rank bows first and lowest.

What should I do if someone ignores my handshake?

Gently drop your hand back to your side. Many different cultural preferences and sensitivities affect the handshake. For example, in the Hindu culture, contact between men and women is avoided, and men do not shake hands with women. There also may be physical limitations or sickness issues.

Is business card etiquette different around the world?

Yes. If you'll be traveling in a foreign country for business, do some research on business card etiquette before leaving home.

As mentioned, people in some countries, such as Germany, are impressed by education and like to see all degrees and titles above the bachelor's degree. In Saudi Arabia, the card should be printed in English on one side and Arabic on the other. When traveling to Poland, bring plenty of cards and give one to everyone you meet (Pagana, K. D., 2006d).

Business cards should be presented with the content face up and readable, but you will find many variations associated with presenting business cards when you are traveling internationally. For example, in China, hold the card with both hands when offering it. In India, the right hand presents and receives the card. In Japan, business cards are given with one hand, but received with both hands (Pagana, K. D., 2007a).

Conversations and Networking

What topics of conversation should I avoid in my travels?

Avoid discussing religion and politics. It is easy to offend people with what may seem like a harmless remark. If someone tries to engage you in a conversation about politics or religion, say something like, "I've learned never to discuss politics or religion." Then change the subject. For example, ask about a cultural landmark.

Are there any American expressions, jargon, or idioms to avoid?

Yes. Even if the person understands and speaks English, he or she may be confused by certain expressions. If you say something and get a confused look, think of another way of saying it. Listed below are some examples of phrases that do not translate well.

- ASAP

- Twenty-four-seven (24/7)

- Shoot yourself in the foot

- Take your foot out of your mouth

- It's a double-header

- Think outside the box

- Hit the ground running

- Dead as a doornail

Should I be concerned about using gestures?

Yes. Several gestures can be misunderstood or considered insulting. Here are some examples of gestures to avoid:

- The OK sign (making a circle with the thumb and forefinger and having three raised fingers) is offensive in many countries, such as Brazil. It means *money* in Japan and means *worthless* in France (Pachter, 2013).

- The thumbs up sign is considered rude in Egypt.

- The V for victory sign, especially with the palm facing inward, is offensive in Great Britain and Canada.

- Pointing or snapping your fingers is offensive in many countries.

- Waving your hand with your arm raised may be misunderstood to mean *no*.

Is it considered friendly to use first names when traveling?

No. This informality is common in the United States, but it will probably be considered disrespectful when traveling abroad. Instant familiarity usually does not make a good impression in other parts of the world. Never begin using first names until given permission (but be aware you may never be given permission). Address people by their proper titles. Titles such as *doctor* and *professor* are highly valued in Germany, Italy, and many other countries (Whitmore, 2005).

TIP

In general, businesspeople should follow the customs of the country they are in.

How do I know how much eye contact is appropriate?

Investigate this. In the United States, people are encouraged to look into the eyes of the person with whom they are communicating. In many Asian countries, however, looking away is a sign of respect. In France, you may be looked at more intently than you expect (Pachter, 2013; Purnell, 2012).

How can I develop effective relationships in a business setting?

The American business practice of "getting right down to business" is not shared by other cultures. Do not expect other cultures to do business the American way.

Instead, focus on relationships. Don't try to push past relationship building to get to business. The "getting to know you" phase builds trust. Executives in regions such as Asia, Latin America, and the Middle East place a premium on relationship protocol. In Japan, for example, you may be invited for tea several times before someone decides whether to do business with you (Whitmore, 2005).

How do I handle personal space issues when traveling?

Handle this with care. Be aware that proximity when conversing with someone is dictated by custom. The average U.S. distance is approximately 3 feet. In Italy and Argentina, it's closer. In Japan, it's farther away (Pachter, 2013; Pagana, K. D., 2013a).

What key etiquette ideas can I learn by observation?

You can learn how people treat each other, act, and dress by being alert and watching those around you. For example, in some cultures, you should not put your hands on your lap during a meal. Notice if people rest their wrists on the edge of the table.

Notice how a diner signals for the waitstaff. If you do not understand why something is done, it is OK to ask. If you do not know what utensil you should use at a meal, follow the example of the native host or guest.

A traveler of taste will notice that the wise are polite all over the world, but the fool only at home.

–Oliver Goldsmith

Should I accept social invitations when on business in another country?

Yes. If you are invited somewhere, go and enjoy the experience. You will get a better understanding of the culture. If the invitation is to a home, be sure to bring a gift for the host. If you refuse an invitation, your host may feel insulted. That can have a negative impact on your business relationship.

✓ **Good Idea!**

Anita traveled with her family to the Ukraine and met many relatives. She was surprised at dinner when a large bowl of soup was placed in the center of the table and everyone was given a spoon. Although she wanted to ask for her own bowl, she followed the example of her hosts. That is the kind of flexibility and tolerance needed for traveling abroad.

Dining and Drinking Etiquette

What are some differences in dining etiquette?

This is a key area for research before getting to your destination. Many business discussions take place over a meal. You don't want to be caught off guard with your actions or your expressions. Here are some examples (Pagana, K. D., 2013b):

- You may have to sit on the floor and eat with your hands.

- You may be served food that looks slimy or has eyes. You may offend your host if you do not eat the food.

- Observe how people ask for more food and how they signal when they have had enough. For example, in Thailand, leaving food on your plate means you are finished and the food was delicious. In Cambodia, cleaning your plate means you still want more food. In Japan, cleaning your plate means you appreciate the food (Whitmore, 2005).

- Don't comment on table manners. Be aware of your nonverbal expressions. Good table manners vary from country to country. For example, making a slurping noise while eating is acceptable to the Japanese (Pachter, 2013).

- Mealtimes vary. If you are the visitor, you must adapt. For example, in Spain, the dinner hour is usually much later than 7:00 p.m.

- It is proper etiquette to remain standing until shown where to sit. For example, in Japan, an honored guest sits at the center of the table farthest from the door and begins eating first.

- In some countries, such as Germany, you may see people cutting food with a fork. This compliments the chef by showing the food is tender.

You can learn a lot by observing and following the actions of the hosts.

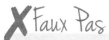
X Faux Pas

When Justin was traveling in the Middle East, he was a guest at a large banquet. Each time he finished eating his food—when he "cleaned his plate"—he was served another helping. Because the server wanted to be polite, he kept adding food to Justin's plate. Justin finally learned that when you are finished eating, you should leave food on your plate.

What should I do if I am the guest of honor in a foreign country and am served an unknown local delicacy?

Try the food. If you leave it on your plate without trying it, you may insult your host. In some cases, your host may wait for you to take a bite before he or she begins. Keep in mind that in many countries, acceptance of food and drinks implies acceptance of the host.

Only ask about a particular food or what is in a particular meal if you have allergies or need to be on a special diet. Be prepared to communicate this information in a clear and respectful manner. If possible, try to communicate dietary restrictions before the meal.

If I am hosting a dinner for international visitors, what foods are considered taboo?

Check this out before you plan the meal. You can ask the person if there are any foods that he or she does not eat. This consideration is very important and demonstrates respect for other cultures. For example, Muslims and Jews do not eat pork, Hindus do not eat beef.

Carry hand sanitizer with you. Not all bathrooms have soap.

What about drinking alcohol?

Don't consume too much. Observe and respect the local customs. In some areas, you will be encouraged to drink. For example, drinking wine is an important part of a European meal.

If you drink, be smart about it. If you do not drink alcohol, have a soda with a lime or lemon. Note that it is against religious principles to drink alcohol in many Middle Eastern countries. Don't drink if your host does not drink.

Tim invited a colleague from the hospital and that colleague's spouse to his home for dinner. The couple was from Turkey. Tim's wife made her dinner specialty: flank steak rolled up with pieces of bacon. Unfortunately, the guests could not eat the meat because of the bacon.

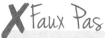 Faux Pas

An American college professor was traveling with a group of students in London. One evening, before leaving a pub, she paid the bill and left a tip. A few minutes later, the bartender handed her a piece of paper with a time and his address. He assumed the tip was a proposition! Her students enjoyed telling that story at home.

Gift Giving

How do I know if I need a gift?

Gift-giving customs are tricky and need to be researched. For example, expensive gifts in China may be considered a bribe. In the Middle East, gifts are exchanged with the right hand because the left hand is used for hygiene.

If you are dining at someone's home, you should bring a gift for the host. In some countries, the host expects a business gift. For example, gifts are expected in Japan, but not in Germany.

How can I give the right gift?

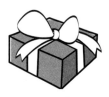

Research gift-giving customs ahead of time. It is hard to go wrong with nice pens, chocolates, toys for children, local crafts from your area, or illustrated books from your country.

Sometimes, a gift can have a negative meaning. Here are some examples to avoid:

- **China:** A clock is associated with funerals.

- **England:** White lilies are only for funerals.

- **Germany:** Red flowers are only for lovers.

- **Saudi Arabia:** Alcohol is illegal.

- **Mexico:** Yellow flowers symbolize death.

How do I know when I should open a gift?

Etiquette dictates whether or not to open a gift in another country. Keep these points in mind:

- In China, it is inappropriate to open a gift when you receive it. By not opening it, you show that the giving of the gift is more valuable than the actual item (Pachter, 2013).

- In some cultures, such as South Korea, the gift initially will not be accepted. Be persistent, because the refusal is part of the ritual.

- In Muslim countries, your left hand is considered unclean. Do not give a gift with your left hand.

- In Japan, gift giving is a refined art with many symbolic meanings. It is best to seek guidance from an advisor or a Japanese friend. For example, gifts should be wrapped in lightly tinted paper, not white paper, as it symbolizes death. They should be given and received with both hands. They will be opened after the gift-giver has departed.

Social Taboos

What are some social taboos I should be aware of?

The following examples will give you an idea of the wide variety of potential faux pas that can occur with international travel. You will see blunders related to communication, body language, gestures, personal space, and dining. Use these guidelines to develop awareness and to serve as a starting point for your country-specific research. This information will enable you to present yourself in the best light possible.

Argentina

- It is rude to yawn in public or eat while walking down the street.

- Placing your hands on your hips is interpreted as a challenge.

- Don't put your feet up on any furniture.

Australia

- Do not imitate Australians by saying "G'day, mate" instead of "hello." It may be perceived as patronizing.

Canada

- The V for victory sign is perceived as an insult when flashed with the palm inward.

- In some areas, it is bad manners to eat while walking down the street.

- Don't be boastful.

China

- Don't ignore the importance of rank in your business relationships. Keep this in mind during all communications.

- Don't use large hand movements. Chinese people do not talk with their hands and may find this distracting.

- Don't point when speaking.

France

- Don't walk down the street greeting people and smiling. Many Americans are friendly and smile easily as an expression of happiness. In Paris, people will think you are crazy (Steves, 2013)!

- Don't speak in a loud voice in a restaurant.

- Don't wear overpowering or glitzy jewelry or other objects.

Germany

- Never place a business call to a person's home. Family and business are kept separate.

- The OK sign is considered obscene.

- Keep your hands out of your pockets.

- Don't wave or call out a person's name in a public place.

- Don't chew gum while talking to someone.

- Punctuality is the norm and is expected.

Great Britain

- Avoid the expression "What do you do?" In Great Britain, inquiring about a person's livelihood is considered intrusive and rude.

- Don't talk business at social events.

- Men should wear shoes with laces, not loafers.

Hong Kong

- If your colleague is silent, don't jump in and start talking. Silence is a form of communication in many Asian cultures.

Italy

- Don't exchange business cards at social events. Hold them for business functions.

- Don't expect quick decisions or actions. The bureaucracy is slow.

- Don't talk about politics or World War II.

Japan

- Avoid physical contact after the initial handshake.

- Don't look people directly in the eye. It invades their privacy.

- Never boast. A self-effacing manner is preferred.

- Never say "no" or "I can't do it." The Japanese prefer not to use the word no. This can confuse negotiations.

Mexico

- Mexicans like to get close. It is rude to pull away when talking.

- Keep your hands out of your pockets.

- Don't stand with your hands on your hips. This suggests aggressiveness.

Poland

- Avoid shouting. Poles speak softly.

- Don't put your hands on your lap when dining. Keep your hands above the table.

Russia

- Don't ignore age, rank, or position. Hierarchy is very important. The most senior person generally makes the decision.

Saudi Arabia

- The thumbs up sign is considered rude.

- Don't discuss religion, politics, or sex.

- Don't pull away if a Saudi colleague embraces you or holds your hand.

- Never show bare shoulders, stomach, calves, or thighs.

- Never show the bottoms of your feet.

- Don't eat with the left hand. It is considered unclean and used for hygiene.

Turkey

- Don't cross your legs or show the soles of your shoes.

- Show respect to elders. Shake hands with the oldest person first.

- Stand when an older person enters the room.

- Don't cross your arms when facing someone.

- Keep your hands out of your pockets.

Venezuela

- Avoid being too attentive to someone of the opposite sex. Your intentions may be misconstrued (Post, 2014).

- Avoid slouching when seated.

- Don't dominate the conversation. Venezuelans like to be in control.

Where can I get information on things like gift-giving customs, restaurants, hotels, social expectations, and cultural taboos?

Here are some valuable resources:

- *Kiss, Bow, or Shake Hands: The Bestselling Guide to Doing Business in More Than 60 Countries* by T. Morrison and W. A. Conaway (Adams Media)

- Executive Planet (www.executiveplanet.com)

- International Business Etiquette and Manners for Global Travelers (www.cyborlink.com)

- International Business Etiquette (http://visual.ly/international-business-etiquette)

- Guidebooks, such as Fodor's, Frommer's, Lonely Planet, and Rick Steves

- Phone apps that provide information about different countries

Travel Safety

How can I ensure my safety, especially when traveling alone?

Here are some suggestions:

- Don't be taken by surprise. Always be alert.

- Appearing timid or scared makes you look like a victim. Walk with confidence. Don't look like a victim.

- Bring maps.

- Avoid walking in alleys or deserted areas.

- At night, walk in well-lit areas.

- Only visit ATMs during the day (Rickenbacher, 2004).

- Choose an ATM in a busy public place.

Is it safe to use local transportation?

It may be safer to travel with the locals. Pickpockets and terrorists may not target local buses as much as tourist buses. Local transportation is a great way to get a feel for the culture of a country. You get to see what the local people wear and talk about (if you can understand them).

Local transportation may not be your best option if you need to get somewhere by a certain time. Frequent stopping results in slower travel (Pagana, T. N., 2008).

How can I avoid being a pickpocket target?

Look confident and goal-oriented, even if you are lost or nervous. Use a money belt to keep your passport and money hidden. Keep expensive electronic gadgets or jewelry out of sight and away from easy-access pockets. It is a good idea to leave these items at home so you won't worry about them getting lost or stolen (Pagana, T. N., 2008).

See the following list for common scams that can distract you and make you a victim of a pickpocket (Steves, 2013):

- A young woman carrying a baby trips and falls into you. While helping her up, she steals your wallet or purse.

TIP

Pickpockets regularly work in churches. Be on your guard at all times.

- Someone approaches you and asks you to help with a demonstration. The person makes a friendship bracelet on your arm. When finished, you are asked to pay for the bracelet.

- An innocent-looking person picks up a ring off the ground and asks if the "gold ring" belongs to you. When you say no, they offer to sell it for a good price. While you are distracted, a nearby and unnoticed partner-in-crime grabs your wallet or purse and runs off.

- Someone asks you if you speak English. When you say yes, they ask you to sign a petition. While you are signing, they grab your valuables.

What should I do if I am approached by a potential scammer?

Say "no" in a firm voice and walk away. Don't smile and don't apologize.

What should I do if I am lost?

Don't panic. Go inside somewhere safe. Then look at your map or ask someone for help. Avoid looking confused while out in a public area. It may make you an easy target for thieves (Pagana, T. N., 2008).

TIP

If you feel unsafe, follow your intuition and remove yourself from the situation.

What should I do if I have an emergency?

In case of an emergency, contact the United States embassy or consulate immediately. You should be sure you have the location and contact information for the embassy or consulate before you leave home. (See www.usembassy.gov for a list of embassies worldwide.) If you need the number of an English-speaking doctor, the consulate can give you one. If you get in trouble with the police, the consulate can help you.

Frequently Asked Questions

(?) Can I use the American style of dining when traveling in Europe?

Yes. Be aware, however, that almost everyone else will be using the Continental style of dining.

(?) What should I do if I lose my passport in a foreign country?

Report your loss to the nearest U.S. embassy or consulate or to the local police. It is easier to replace a passport if you have a photocopy of the data page. If you are traveling with someone, give him or her a copy of your passport. It is also a good idea to have a scanned version of your passport available via webmail or online in some other location that you can access if you need to.

(?) How do I know if I need a visa for traveling abroad?

Call the consulate or embassy of the country you want to visit.

(?) If I do not understand why someone does something in a certain way, is it OK to ask him or her?

Yes. Polite questions show you have an interest in another culture. This will help build relationships.

(?) Is it OK to use humor when conversing with people abroad?

It is better not to use humor because humor is subjective. Some jokes do not translate well and could cause offense or confusion.

Is it acceptable to wear native clothing when attending a business meeting in another country?

No. This is inappropriate unless encouraged by your hosts.

 Is it appropriate to help myself to the food at a business meal?

No. Helping yourself is an American custom. Wait until food is offered.

 When traveling out of the country, is gift giving a nice touch?

Gift giving is expected in some countries. Find this out before you travel. Also learn what gifts are appropriate.

 I am planning a trip to Japan. Should I learn how to use chopsticks?

Yes. Learn and practice using them before you travel. Don't point with them. Don't pierce food with them. When you are taking a break to drink or talk, rest them on the chopstick rest.

 Where should I put my hands when dining?

In America, it is OK to place your hands on your lap. However, in many countries, such as France and Poland, the hands are kept above the table. It is inappropriate to put them on your lap.

 Can I use my cell phone while traveling abroad?

Before you travel, check with your cell-phone provider. You should be able to purchase a travel plan for a short period of time. Find out about calling and data charges so you do not end up with unexpected high charges.

TAKE-AWAY TIPS

✓ Think of international travel as an adventure, an opportunity, and a learning experience.

✓ The old adage "When in Rome, do as the Romans do" is true.

✓ Respect cultural differences.

✓ Notify your credit card companies prior to travel.

✓ If possible, avoid changing money at airports, where it is more expensive. Instead, use a local bank or ATM.

✓ Don't brag about American culture. This is rude.

✓ It is not acceptable to make a mistake and simply say, "I didn't know."

✓ Refrain from using first names without prior permission.

✓ The American way isn't the only way—nor is it always the best way.

Test Your Knowledge

1. When someone compliments you, you should find a way to return the compliment.

   True   False

2. The proper placement for your name tag is over your heart.

   True   False

3. It is polite to ask permission before writing on someone's business card.

   True   False

4. Sending a thank-you note for a gift by email is perfectly acceptable.

   True   False

5. Where would you find your water glass?

   To the right of the entrée plate   To the left of the entrée plate

6. What should you do if someone repeatedly mispronounces your name?

   Relax, let it go, and ignore   Help that person find a way
   the mispronunciation.   to remember how to
                                           pronounce it.

7. Whose name should you mention first when introducing your new staff nurse to your supervisor?

Staff nurse   Supervisor

8. You should not schedule a meeting if your goals can be accomplished through email.

True   False

9. When traveling internationally and dining at the home of your host, you can't go wrong by bringing flowers as a gift.

True   .   False

10. You should be cautious using the blind carbon copy (BCC) feature because the practice can be considered deceptive.

True   False

11. If you need to excuse yourself during a meal, you should fold your napkin and place it to the right of your plate.

True   False

12. Talking about your children is not always a safe conversational topic when meeting people at a business cocktail party.

True   False

13. When signing up for social media accounts, it doesn't matter whether you use your personal or work email.

True   False

14. When networking at a nursing conference, you should pass out your business cards to as many people as you can.

   True   False

15. You should not embarrass your co-worker by telling her that she has poppy seeds in her teeth.

   True   False

16. Dressing professionally is more of a challenge for women than for men.

   True   False

17. It is best to arrive 10 to 15 minutes early for a meeting.

   True   False

18. Websites are easier to create and update than blogs.

   True   False

19. Placing silverware in the finished position signals to the wait-staff that your plate can be removed.

   True   False

20. If the hotel desk clerk makes your room number public, you should ask for another room.

   True   False

Quiz Answers

1. False. The best way to handle a compliment is to smile and say, "Thank you." Don't feel compelled to return the compliment. Always be sincere when complimenting someone.

2. False. Place your name tag on the right side of your chest so it can be easily seen when shaking hands.

3. True. In some parts of the world, the business card is viewed as a representation of the owner. You deface the card if you write on it without permission.

4. False. When you receive a gift, take the time to show your appreciation by writing a thank-you note.

5. Your water glass and all glasses and cups to the right of the entrée plate belong to you.

6. If someone repeatedly mispronounces your name, help that person find a way to remember the correct pronunciation. For example, "Mallon" is pronounced like "Gallon."

7. Your supervisor's name is mentioned first because he or she is the senior person.

8. True. If people don't need to be physically present, don't schedule a meeting. This shows respect for people's time.

9. False. Some flowers have negative meanings. For example, in Mexico, yellow flowers symbolize death. In England, white lilies are only for funerals. When traveling abroad, choosing the right host gift requires a little research.

10. True. Only use the BCC feature when sending emails to people who don't know each other to protect their privacy. This also keeps all recipients anonymous.

11. False. During a meal, place your napkin on your chair when you excuse yourself.

12. True. Be sensitive to the fact that some people may not be able to have children. Don't monopolize the conversation talking about your brilliant children.

13. False. It is better to use your personal account. Using your work email address may violate your workplace's social media policy. In addition, you may receive distracting notification about personal matters during work hours.

14. False. Wait to be asked for your business card. Usually, if you ask others for a card, they will ask you for your card.

15. False. People want to know this and will appreciate your thoughtfulness.

16. True. Men know they look professional when they wear a suit and tie. The leeway in defining professional dress for women leads to the potential for inappropriate clothing.

17. False. You can create an awkward situation if you arrive early and those in charge are still ironing out last-minute details for the meeting.

18. False. Blogs are easily created and updated without needing technical expertise.

19. True. To indicate that you are finished, place the knife and fork in the 10 and 4 o'clock position with the tops of the silverware pointed at 10 and the bottoms pointed at 4.

20. True. Keeping your room number private is an important safety issue, especially when traveling alone.

References

Adubato, S. (2005). *Make the connection: Improve your communication at work and at home.* Piscataway, NJ: Rutgers University Press.

Brody, M. (2005). *Professional impressions: Etiquette for everyone, every day* (3rd ed.). Jenkintown, PA: Career Skills Press.

Brown, R. E., & Johnson, D. A. (2004). *The power of handshaking.* Sterling, VA: Capital Books.

Candiotti, S., & Duke, A. (2014, November 11). Source: Joan Rivers' doctor took selfie, began biopsy before her cardiac arrest. *CNN.* Retrieved from http://www.cnn.com/2014/09/16/showbiz/joan-rivers-clinic/index.html?sr=sharebar_twitter

Chaney, L. H., & Martin, J. S. (2007). *The essential guide to business etiquette.* Westport, CT: Praeger Publications.

Clark, C. (2013). *Creating & sustaining civility in nursing education.* Indianapolis, IN: Sigma Theta Tau International Honor Society of Nursing.

DelBalzo, J. (2014). The social media etiquette guide to business (infographic). *Business 2 Community.* Retrieved from http://www.business2community.com/infographics/social-media-etiquette-infographic-2-01021902

Fox, S. (2007). *Business etiquette for dummies* (2nd ed.). New York, NY: Wiley Publishing.

Gould, C. (2014, August 19). Etiquette tip of the week: Breaking bread at a breakfast meeting. *Des Moines Register.* Retrieved from http://blogs.desmoinesregister.com/dmr/index.php/2014/08/19/etiquette-tip-of-the-week-breaking-bread-at-a-breakfast-meeting/article

Headley, C. M. (2007). Keeping your elbows off your career table. *Nephrology Nursing Journal, 34*(3), 357–358.

Kintish, W. (2006). *I hate networking! Discover the secrets of confident and effective networkers.* Manchester, Ontario, Canada: JAM Publications.

Krames, J. A. (2002). *The Rumsfeld way: Leadership wisdom of a battle-hardened maverick.* New York, NY: McGraw-Hill.

Liburdi, M. C. (2008). Working it!: How to make the most out of social networking to enhance career prospects. *NSNA Imprint, 55*(4), 62–70.

Lower, J. (2007). Creating a culture of civility in the workplace: Use these 7 challenges to clean up a toxic work environment. *American Nurse Today, 2*(9), 49–52.

Mitchell, M. (2004). *The complete idiot's guide to etiquette* (3rd ed.). Indianapolis, IN: Alpha Books.

National Safety Council. (2014). NSC releases latest injury and fatality statistics and trends. *National Safety Council.* Retrieved from http://www.nsc.org/NewsDocuments/2014-Press-Release-Archive/3-25-2014-Injury-Facts-release.pdf

Pachter, B. (2013). *The essentials of business etiquette: How to greet, eat, and tweet your way to success.* New York, NY: McGraw Hill Education.

Pagana, K. D. (2005a, July). Dining etiquette: A necessary ingredient for the true professional. *Create the Future Through Renewal, 2*(6).

Pagana, K. D. (2005b). Get in good with the gatekeepers: Tips for avoiding business call blunders. *Pharmaceutical Representative, 35*(9), 44–45.

Pagana, K. D. (2006a). Blunder-free business meals. *American Nurse Today, 1*(3), 61–62.

Pagana, K. D. (2006b). *Bread, butter & beyond: Dining etiquette.* Williamsport, PA: LAYCO Publishing.

Pagana, K. D. (2006c). Business etiquette blunders quiz. *Business Credit, 108*(10), 34–35.

Pagana, K. D. (2006d). Do you need a business card? *American Nurse Today*, *1*(2), 47.

Pagana, K. D. (2007a). Business card etiquette: Leaving the right impression. *Networking Times*, *6*(3), 28–29.

Pagana, K. D. (2007b). Crossing your 't's and dotting your 'i's: Professional etiquette in nursing. In C. M. Headley (Ed.), *Career fulfillment in nephrology nursing: Your guide to professional development* (2nd ed.), (pp. 63–74). Pitman, NY: Anthony J. Jannetti.

Pagana, K. D. (2007c). E-mail etiquette: 17 tips for professional communication. *American Nurse Today*, *2*(7), 45.

Pagana, K. D. (2007d). The etiquette advantage: The nurse's toolbox. *Journal of Continuing Education in Nursing*, *38*(3), 105–106.

Pagana, K. D. (2009a). A user's guide to cell phone etiquette. *American Nurse Today*, *4*(3), 36–37.

Pagana, K. D. (2009b). The art of small talk. *Nursing Spectrum & Nurse Week, Nurse.Com. Career Fair Guide*, 60–61.

Pagana, K. D. (2011a). Facebook: Know the policy before posting. *Nurse.com*, *24*(6), 54–59.

Pagana, K. D. (2011b). Voice mail etiquette. *American Nurse Today*, *6*(5), 21–22.

Pagana, K. D. (2012a). Ten tips for handling job interviews by phone. *American Nurse Today*, *7*(1), 40–41.

Pagana, K. D. (2012b). How to keep your communications professional. *American Nurse Today*, *7*(9), 56–58.

Pagana, K. D. (2013a). Making professional connections. *American Nurse Today*, *8*(9), 32–34.

Pagana, K. D. (2013b). Mind your manners...multiculturally. *Nurse.com*. Retrieved from http://ce.nurse.com/course/ce570/mind-your-manners-multiculturally/

Pagana, K. D. (2013c). Ride to the top with a good elevator speech. *American Nurse Today*, *8*(3), 14–17.

Pagana, K. D. (2013d). Social media: Give your career a boost. *Nurse.com*. Retrieved from http://ce.nurse.com/content/ce691/social-media/

Pagana, K. D. (2014). STOP: A strategy for dealing with difficult conversations. *American Nurse Today*, 9(9), 20–21.

Pagana, T. N. (2008). *Tips for the thrifty traveler: How to travel the world cheaply, easily, & safely*. Williamsport, PA: LAYCO Publishing.

Post, P. (2014). *Emily Post's the etiquette advantage in business* (3rd ed.). New York, NY: Harper Collins.

Purnell, L. D. (2012). *Transcultural health care: A culturally competent approach* (4th ed.). Philadelphia, PA: F. A. Davis Co.

Rickenbacher, C. (2004). *Be on your best business behavior*. Dallas, TX: Brown Books.

Sabath, A. (2010). *Business etiquette: 101 ways to conduct business with charm & savvy* (3rd ed.). Franklin Lakes, NJ: Career Press.

Safko, L., & Brake, D. (2009). *The social media bible: Tactics, tools, & strategies for business success*. Hoboken, NJ: John Wiley & Sons.

Saver, C. (2011). Inter- and intra-generational communication. In K. D. Pagana (Ed.), *The nurse's communication advantage: How business-savvy communication can advance your nursing career*. Indianapolis, IN: Sigma Theta Tau International Honor Society.

Schindler, E. (2008, February 15). Running an effective teleconference or virtual meeting [Web log post]. *CIO.com*. Retrieved from http://www.cio.com/article/2437139/collaboration/running-an-effective-teleconference-or-virtual-meeting.html

Scott, D. M. (2009). *The new rules of marketing and PR*. Hoboken, NJ: John Wiley & Sons.

Shipley, D., & Schwalbe, W. (2007). *Send: The essential guide to e-mail for office and home*. New York, NY: Alfred A. Knopf.

Smolenski, M. C. (2002, November). Playing the credentials game. *Nursing Spectrum*. Retrieved from http://www.pdflibrary.org/pdf/playing-the-credentials-game-mary-c-smolenski-edd-fnp.html

Spade, K. (2004). *Manners: Always gracious, sometimes irreverent.* New York, NY: Simon & Schuster.

Steves, R. (2013). *Rick Steves' Paris 2014.* Berkeley, CA: Avalon Travel.

Tocco, S., & DeFontes, J. (2014). Managing our fears to improve patient safely. *American Nurse Today, 9*(5), 34–38.

University Alliance. (n. d.) Social media for nurses: guidelines and policies. *Villanova University.* Retrieved from http://www.villanovau.com/resources/nursing/social-media-guidelines-for-nurses/#.VQWzNPnF9rU

Vance, C. (2011). *Fast facts for career success in nursing: Making the most of mentoring in a nutshell.* New York, NY: Springer Publishing Co.

Whitmore, J. (2005). *Business class: Etiquette essentials for success at work.* New York, NY: St. Martin's Press.

Index

G

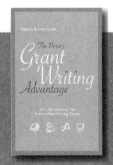
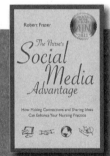
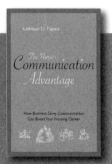
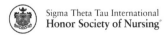
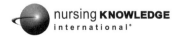

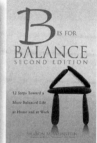
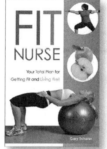
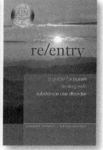
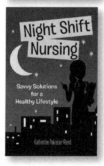

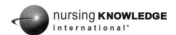

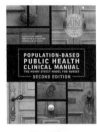
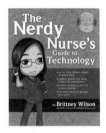
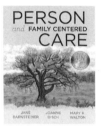
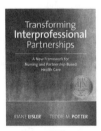
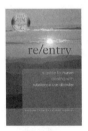
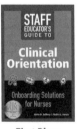
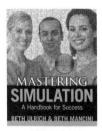
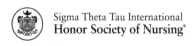
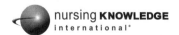